i

# Neogenesis

August Dunning

This book contains the opinions and ideas of its author. It is intended to provide helpful and informative information on the subject discussed herein. It is sold with the understanding that the author is not engaged in rendering medical, health or any other kind of professional services.

This book contains advice and information related to health care. It should be used to supplement rather than replace the advice of your doctor or another trained health professional. The reader should always consult his or her health care provider to determine the appropriateness of the information for his or her own situation or if he or she has any questions regarding a medical condition or treatment plan. It is recommended that you seek your physician's advice before embarking on any medical program or treatment.

All efforts have been made to assure the accuracy of the information contained in this book. The author disclaims any liability for any medical outcomes that may occur as a result of applying the methods suggested in this book.

# Neogenesis

The deliberate activation of cyclical metabolic
regeneration processes to extend
youth-like cellular functionality.

In effect, a process of Functional Immortality

# Neogenesis

# Contents

# Neogenesis

*"When I made my theory of the origin of life it was accepted by everyone except the 'experts', which is quite normal for revolutionary ideas."*

*-Freeman Dyson*

# Neogenesis

**Prologue**... *Becoming unlocked in time*

*I think I see something from the field of medicine that is already working albeit for a singular outcome – the return to health from illness.*

> *"The real voyage of discovery consists not in seeking new landscapes but in having new eyes."*
>
> *-Marcel Proust*

*I, however, see this therapy through new eyes and predict quite a different outcome, one beyond just health if you ask "what if you apply the regenerative benefits of this therapy... if you are not ill?*

> *"The hardest thing to explain is the glaringly evident that everybody has decided not to see."*
>
> *-Ayn Rand*

*Neogenesis is an insight. It manipulates existing metabolic and regeneration systems in a way not thought of before - in a deliberate act to extend lifespan - in a way neither can produce in and of themselves. I think our currently accepted ideas about aging is shockingly incomplete. I would suggest that it is so far out-of-whack that many of the modern illnesses are, at their foundation due to 'user error'.*

*I'll endeavor to make what I now see obvious to you but let me state at the very beginning that Neogenesis only relates what I have discovered and used to reverse aging.*

*'Reverse aging' is admittedly too broad a brush and it's better said: 'what I did to restore tissue and cellular function in a way to measure the restoration of youthful function'. I won't make the same mistake as Eos; asking Zeus to grant eternal life for Tithonus while forgetting to include eternal youth. Let*

# Neogenesis

me be very clear that this book is not about everlastingness; I reject that outcome outright; becoming older and older. It assumes that physical aging is strictly a chronological phenomenon, not a condition representing physical status from repeated neglect or negligence over time.

I seem to be going in the right direction with my experiment.

Here is my personal test result reflecting how my DNAge genetic age is 66, three years lower than my chronological age of 69, as one measure of 'restoring youth by restoring youthful function'

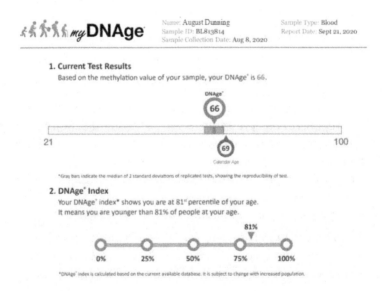

I took this test after my second 7-day dry fast. Unfortunately, I did not take one of these tests before I started dry fasting. I can only imagine I would have tested significantly older genetically due to my earlier sedentary positions with years of laboratory time plus I ate fast-food and had never exercised. Paradoxically, several online health influencers', that have channels presenting their rigorous regimes of exercise and diet for anti-aging, also performed the same DNAge test. To their consternation they were older genetically than their chronological age. To my knowledge none of them have performed dry fasting. I suspect that this is the difference between mine and their results.

Ironically, most of us do some things from a long list of diet, exercise, and cleansing practices just by 'chance' or habit and live a bit healthier and a bit longer...a bit...not a lot.

**Why after all this time has research not figured this 'life length' thing out?**
Maybe our time alive may just be by luck. Lifespan may only be the time it takes to wear out the body by never cleaning and repairing it. But indeed, there are no magic pills or bullets, yet Neogenesis may be a first step to put as many of these 'chances' in a row, in a morning, in a day, week, month...or for good to achieve a type of functional immortality.
I know, I know; it's a far-fetched idea - functional immortality. It can easily be derided like the Stephen Wright joke...

**"I've decided to live forever...so far, so good..."**

But seen with a set of 'new eyes' one might see something 'glaringly evident' if presented with the right data. So, I decided some sort of guide might be a good start or at least a record of my successes.

We've tried endless applications of therapies to address aging but even Hippocrates said "to do nothing is sometimes the best medicine"; how prophetic as you will see.

# Neogenesis

*Moreover, after reading this book, I hope you grasp what happens if you don't implement some of the ideas herein and take care of the excellent vessel your mother birthed.*

*Our current pathetically short lifespan that ends too soon and typically in a nursing home might be a correctable error resulting from a missing user's manual. That's why I wrote this book.*

*I don't want to achieve old age I want continual youth – I want more 'now'.*

*The future is a projection, the past dies as we move through time, the only moment that matters is right now. 'Now' is my battle ground.*

*To that end this book is not focused on everlastingness, it is instead very sharply focused on...ever-presence.*

*August – 2021*

## Many, Many Questions

*"As you get older the questions come down
to about two or three. How long do I have?
What do I do with the time I have left?"*

-David Bowie

# Neogenesis

**Why have we seen no dramatic leaps in lifespan yet?**
Living a dramatically extended lifespan in a youthful, supple, strong body is a goal that STILL eludes us because, perhaps, we have run off into a box canyon of thinking.

**I think this is what we've missed:**
The healing and regenerative actions of extending the sleep cycle <aka> dry fasting, to provide a level of autophagy normal sleep cannot, combined with exercise and amino acid focused nutrition during the eating cycle, should result in an improved cellular metabolism and the structural repair that we seek to extend lifespan; that neither alone can provide in and of themselves.

> *"Detoxification is more important that nutrition."*
> *-David Wolfe*

**The missing piece of the puzzle**
It's my opinion that the puzzle of radical life extension has never been solved because the focus has only been on the eating cycle by applying foods, drugs, therapies and even manipulating the eating cycle itself. Calorie restriction, intermittent fasting, OMAD, and even the fasting mimicking diet can't achieve dry fasting's ability to remove decades of stored intercellular toxins that act to shorten life. They simply can't work because all these regimes still involve eating.

*As a side note, whereas water fasting doesn't involve eating, it does involve drinking and to that extent it doesn't create endogenous water that can flush the cells from the inside out. Hence, water fasting doesn't remove the intercellular 'slag' that is removed during a dry fast simply because you are still drinking.*

It's now obvious that none of these ideas have extended lifespan. And like any puzzle with a missing piece, life extension experts have never considered this missing piece; the benefits of extending the sleep cycle.

**This is why I think we haven't seen any dramatic leaps in lifespan.**

### Is life extension youth extension?

Young blood plasma transfusions (from donors 16 to 25) have recently been touted as the 'fountain of youth'. The transfusions are designed to replace proteins no longer found in older peoples' blood. This apparently worked well in mice, but I'll pass. It all seems a bit too vampiric to me but if seen with new eyes it's proof of an idea I've been knocking around for months. Until right now as you read this, never in human history has the following glaringly evident view of aging ever been considered:

> "What if young people are 'young' only because
> they are living in a young body?"

I know, it sounds absurd, but a 'young' body has a significantly higher level of osteocalcin (more on that later), lower or no amount of epigenetic methylation tags that reduce protein code access, low levels of pathogenic organisms and parasites, less senescent

9

cells and their cytokines and much less advanced glycosylated end products compared to an adult who has all this metabolic baggage. Not to mention a young body has less of the 50,000+ different man-made chemical 'agents of aging' common to the modern biosphere most adults have accumulated. It's a global health disaster, microplastics have even made it to the Arctic and Antarctic.

**"We don't face a climate crisis;
we face a habitat crisis."**

Young body cells haven't lived long enough to need system wide cellular repair or replacement because not enough time has passed to accumulate enough toxins to wreak system wide damage; the ticking time bomb around humanity's neck, burdening us metabolically more and more, each passing day.

As I said in the Phoenix protocol:

> *"Youth is not measured in years
> it's measured in functionality".*

Another guy said it this way:

> *"In order to radically extend lifespan
> ...we must stay younger longer".*
>
> *-Aubrey DeGray*

'Just stay younger longer'...hmm...a novel approach to life extension Aubrey, to be sure but...uh...how exactly is that achieved? And how much will it cost?

I have some ideas of how to achieve this but moreover, it's those ideas that are not only easy to understand but also easy to adopt that usually have a chance to be passed along.

I think this book provides ample evidence that the idea (*that we can purposely turn on innate anti-aging regeneration systems*) is sound and that getting into and staying in good health and physical shape is far easier than anyone thought. It doesn't take expensive equipment like 620nm red light grid system walls or gene therapy. It only requires knowing what we really are and what we already have available to us after millions of years of evolution. The 'message' in Neogenesis is simple: stay trim and strong with good bone density by eating genetically recognizable, non-chemically soaked food, timed with exercise.

**Ideas that work are obvious**
Toward the end of writing The Phoenix Protocol, I started to see overall beneficial bio-physical changes that accelerated when I started lifting weights and focusing on amino acids to target specific types of tissue in my body, my tendons. This repaired a 50-year-old shoulder injury, from a bicycle accident in college, in only a few months. This led me to view the body we inhabit very differently.

**How differently?**
Our perception of the world only begins at the skin. Skin is a tough outer membrane covering a vast network of specific proteins, collagen, and proteoglycan filaments.

# Neogenesis

Our body is a genetically patterned matrix of protein membrane compartments and webbing that encapsulates everything else inside the skin like the skeleton, muscles, organs, heart, and brain utilizing a tension / compression architecture that allows us to walk upright. This pervasive fibrous network is connected to the brain with sensors that monitor the internal and external environment. This protein matrix has very special characteristics from adapting to ancient drought and famine that allows for species survival. We can still survive significant periods of starvation for example.

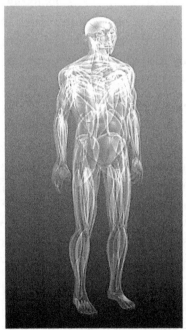

**The Fascial Matrix**

# Neogenesis

This protein architecture, that encapsulates all the body parts and holds all the stem cell reservoirs, was for decades only thought of as 'connective tissue' [41].

**20 different bricks to make an infinite number of walls**
You are a highly evolved and integrated four body protein system with a consciousness; a system of subsystems that has only recently been described as such. Its integration with the micro biome population to maintain stasis as the 'other' you, are an accommodation between the first kingdom of life and the third. I will be discussing that at length as well in a later chapter. The common denominator in this microscopic-interlaced structure are the amino acids. The roles of minerals, factors, and co-factors notwithstanding, life erupts during the interacting systems of complex proteins made from 20 simple amino acids. Each amino has a specific and determined purpose alone and synergistically in combinations. I propose that, because all the integrated parts are protein, there is a way to enable a longer lifespan in a younger body in a very simple way using already in-place, evolutionary created, endogenous regeneration systems.

Neogenesis is the way I am activating these naturally occurring endogenous systems to see if I can make my body too young metabolically to die from old age; a neo-genic protocol that incorporates a yearly session of dry fasting and a protocol for restoring muscularity and bone density for durability during the rest of the year.

**Lessons learned**

If you're not sick, don't stress the body by doing multiple 7-day dry fasts yearly. There's nothing to fix and a 7-day dry fast is an extreme form of hormesis by nutrient stress (starvation) and naturally hard on the body if done too often. What I have learned now, after three years, is that one 7-day dry fast per year is adequate.

I have arrived at this conclusion because during my first two 7-day dry fasts copious amounts of orange colored slag was expelled while subsequent fasts only removed a miniscule amount. So, the most significant detoxification occurs during the first 7-day dry fast. Therefore, I suspect that subsequent yearly dry fasts will be more focused on tissue regeneration, remodeling, and cellular repair because detoxification has already been achieved.

**A perspective of method**

The methods of Neogenesis will yield an unusually interesting 'perspective', a new playing field; achieved only by doing 'nothing' for a couple of weeks of the year and being moderately active for 50 weeks. I expect this will yield a physiological condition normally seen at a much younger age; a perspective produced by methods that seem unconnected.

What I am proposing is a way to produce a condition that has never been accomplished.

# Neogenesis

We, as a species, have never been in the position to live during our adult years without the ever-increasing level of toxic debris that causes chronic low-grade inflammation which reduces cellular and system function. Significant positive benefits come from this.

But there is no doubt that Aubrey is also right; staying younger longer is certainly part of the solution. Knowing how to stay younger has always been the trick.

It should be glaringly obvious that extending life could be as simple as providing the right molecular stimulus with the right molecular fuel.

Simply, you are designed for it.

**Steven Wright:** *"I've decided to live forever...so far, so good..."*

**Heckler:** "Yeah? *How's that workin out for ya?"*

**Steven Wright** *"I dunno yet...ask me in 100 years..."*

# Can We Have More Time?

*"Yes, of course, who has time? Who has time?
But then if we never 'take' time, how can
we ever 'have' time?"*
-The Merovingian-The Matrix

Neogenesis

# 1

## Staying 'Here'

*"To know the answer,
you must first know the question."*
- [ chn t'Gai] *Sarek*

# Neogenesis

**How do we stay 'alive'?**

The human body balances two distinct metabolic processes to maintain life; a metabolism when awake and eating and a metabolism when asleep. When awake, we ingest nutrients that power the body's cellular metabolic chemical systems. This waking chemistry normally produces a calculated amount of tissue damage and metabolic waste. Yet, when sleeping, the body transforms to a metabolism that turns on autophagy to try to repair damage and remove waste. Lifespan is therefore significantly benefitted by the sleeping metabolism.

**Why is the average human lifespan only 78.6 years?**

Lifespan is limited to its current average because the length of time in autophagy during sleep is not long enough to regenerate cellular organelles or remove the most difficult metabolic waste produced by the waking and eating metabolism. This difficult to digest waste and calculated tissue damage accumulates over time and in this way accelerates aging by reducing cellular function. The rate and degree of this accumulation of these 'agents of negative outcomes', determines how rapidly or slowly the body ages. Actual lifespans vary greatly because the accumulation can differ significantly from one person to another.

**How can we stay alive longer than the average lifespan?**

It would seem apparent that we can indeed extend lifespan by spending more time in the repair mode, thereby restoring more damaged cells and tissue while removing more of the waste materials that limit lifespan.

## What then, is aging?
Aging is a tissue and cellular malfunction; a reaction to the accumulated metabolic byproducts and genetic insults created during the waking and eating metabolism. Without some sort of a significant pause in this metabolism, normal aging is unavoidable.

## Is aging avoidable?
The issue is not aging, the issue is not getting 'old'. If I'm right, our body already has the capacity to deliberately switch on various repair and regeneration systems; I suspect most people never know they can flip the switch. Sleep is one of those switches. Sleep is a beneficial period of autophagy used to repair and restore the body. There is a switch that can turn on the sleep metabolism for days.

## Sleeping is regenerative
Not eating and drinking changes our body pH to produce a unique metabolism that encourages flushing out cells and repairing the body. This metabolism, seen during sleep, can be maintained by a therapeutic application of not eating and drinking to extend the time in autophagy from hours to days. This extended period of autophagy is quite different than OMAD or intermittent fasting. It takes 2-3 days of not eating and drinking to turn this switch on. Yet, when turned on, it

can provide all the time required for eliminating the metabolic debris that accumulates from the eating metabolism that cannot be eliminated during a normal nightly period of sleep. In essence, planned periods of dry fasting can provide time enough to take out all the trash and not leave any behind.

Waking and sleeping enact significantly different cellularly processes by the acetylation function in cell mitochondria and nuclei by SIRT3 and SIRT1 seen below.

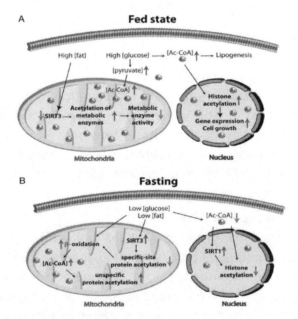

### Dry fasting mimics sleep
Sleep is the body's natural period of no eating and no drinking - anhydrous starvation. The body relies on this non-eating metabolism to make sure there is

uninterrupted excretory and metabolic activity while asleep.

Dry fasting, like sleep, prevents (a) blood hypertonicity (blood concentration of serum sodium), (b) hypovolemia (decreasing volume of blood), and (c) hypoglycemia (deficiency of glucose in the blood) to maintain normal blood pressure, heart rate, and hemoglobin oxygen saturation and assures safe values in serum creatinine, urea, K+, Na+, and plasma glucose. As I described in The Phoenix Protocol, it's the moderate increase in blood borne solids from not drinking that stimulates the hypothalamus and pituitary to release signals to tap fat cells for fuel. Drawing on adipose tissue for fuel insures an abundance of water from fatty acid oxidation in mitochondria for a substantial increase in kidney function as autophagy proceeds [29].

Dry fasting is the perfect way to safely extend sleeps' metabolism to detoxify the system, remove senescent cells, restore old tissue with stem cells, produce a completely new immune system, and restore the functional parts inside and outside cells while mobilizing mitochondria biogenesis.

The Phoenix Protocol is a 7-day dry fast for this reason. It gently starts and maintains ketosis long enough to 'flip a switch' on day 3 to wake up stem cells to replicate and propagate system wide. When the fast is over the body recovers with a lower level of methylation and toxic load.

# Neogenesis

I'm going to show you my way of testing this idea but as Thoreau said, "*not that the story need be long, but it will take a long while to make it short.*"

In this respect it has taken quite some time to extract the most recent scientific discoveries in cellular biology for examples to help you understand why I think we can now radically extend lifespan.

So, from the looks of it, my first book, The Phoenix Protocol, shows how to extend the 'not-eating' metabolism. This book, Neogenesis, covers the 'eating' metabolism. I'm using both to become stronger and progressively more durable. Without strategically utilizing both processes, cleaning, and structural maintenance, we will never exceed what is thought of as the normal human lifespan. You won't have the durability necessary.

The overarching message is this: we can very easily return to our genetically recognizable, non-chemically soaked foods and include simple, and effective physical activity that mimic the environmental stressors that got us here.

We must do this to survive our next great achievement: breaking the time barrier.

# 2

# Breaking the Time Barrier

*"I would just like to really see how long I can last here you know, really in it, really alive in the moment."*

-Bill Murray

# Neogenesis

**What is the possible span of human life?**

I suspect it's longer than we currently think...a lot longer. Because by rarely activating the cleaning metabolism our most widely accepted views of aging may be in serious error. It may have given us a view of lifespan that is spectacularly incomplete. It may prove that the most important reason we even have the lifespan we currently enjoy, as short as it is, is because we sleep. Sleep, a natural period of not eating and drinking, is the only time the body can devote energy to remove metabolic byproducts and chemical toxins as well as repairing the daily damage of living. Normally it's a third of our day and it's universally recognized that *sleep deprivation reduces lifespan*. So perhaps this idea of extending the sleep 'metabolism' while not eating and drinking for extending life is not so farfetched.

**Sleep: natures not-eating metabolism**

No one has considered it until this book but perhaps sleep is enacted by the body not because you are tired but rather is a signal to stop the waste accumulation metabolism and try to remove some of the waste.

Clearly, the non-eating metabolism is poorly understood and how important sleep is for staying alive for as long as we do. But conversely, if you stop eating altogether you most certainly will not live any type of normal human lifespan.

Not surprisingly then, there is a balance between the 'time spent' awake and asleep that has not been fully characterized with respect to its effect on aging.

And yet, a good way to put this is 'Res Ipsa Loquitur'; the legal principle that the occurrence of an accident implies negligence.

Is aging accidental? Is it from user error?

## Metabolic rate

One theory that has been universally accepted at face value is that every species' lifespan is inversely proportional to their characteristic metabolic rate. Yet not having both sides of the coin may have led researchers to arrive at this 'fact' as merely an 'assumption'; that there is a direct relationship of life length and metabolic rate. It's an incomplete view of 'metabolism' without adding in the wide role that sleeping plays.

It is my view that the metabolic rate, as it pertains to lifespan and life, is significantly shortened from many chemical processes that are never turned off or even dialed down for seven to nine decades. The species-wide differences in lifespan might be seen as their metabolic rate verses how long they last if the accumulation of metabolic waste is slower or faster while they continue to eat every day.

And this nonstop daily eating regime produces:

*-Advanced glycated end products in skin, organs, cells, mitochondria, and vascular system.*

*-Environmental and seed oil derived toxins stored in fat cells and organ tissue that destabilize mitochondria.*

-*Senescent cells that don't die yet pump out an unending stream of toxic cytokines that damage adjacent cells and create more parasitic senescent cells that take nutrients but do not add to life force.*

-*Methyl markers left after base excision DNA repair that reduce the amount of accessible protein codes for transcription on histone codes and nuclear DNA.*

-*Indigestible tryptophan metabolites that mimic co-enzyme Q levels that cannot serve as electron doners, subsequently reducing the protection of mitochondria from reactive oxygen species allowing damage to ATP mechanisms that reduce ATP; the 'energy of life'.*

-*Indigestible tyrosine metabolites that neutralize osteocalcin resulting in memory dysfunction, pancreatic dysfunction resulting in fat deposition and testes and ovary dysfunction resulting in reduced fertility, ultimately resulting in sarcopenia.*

## Why is lifespan getting shorter?

Could it be that we are being overwhelmed by the level of toxic chemicals introduced into our biosphere? And what about the exponential rise of stress seen in all societies? Predictably, these factors and many others have a negative effect on lifespan. These challenges added to the ones produced during the 'eating' metabolism: telomere shortening by cell replacement following cellular damage while relying only on sleep to ineffectually address their accumulative damage, well, I think you get the picture. It's overwhelming. This may explain the variations in the time people stay alive as merely the luck of the draw <aka> their level of exposure.

Sometimes later, sometimes earlier but life always ends right around the 78-year average. Obviously reducing these accumulated wastes and stressors or eliminating them altogether will have a positive effect on 'span'.
In fact, the 'signs of aging' are clearly the evidence of the buildup of these impossible to digest metabolites. This situation almost assures an end will arrive sooner than later as the system is packed with toxic debris and unfixed structural damage.

Simply put; the vascular wall linings become too clogged with plaque, calcify, and harden, preventing nutrients to pass into cells throughout the body. Filtration organs: kidneys, liver, lung, and gut are too full of toxins, mitochondria are packed with pathologically remodeled cardiolipin (AGE) reducing ATP production. The reduction in access to essential proteins codes, due to the amount of built-up genetic repair tags, and the overtaxed immune system becomes too overwhelmed for some part or system of the organism to continue the chemical processes of metabolic life.

**Could it be that simple? Yeah! It probably is!**
Seen in this light, the estimated 'normal human lifespan' is just the result of never pausing one metabolism to allow the sub-routine metabolism to operate long enough to clean and restore worn and damaged tissue to maintain youthful function. Habits are important.

# Neogenesis

This could then explain why currently some nutritional and lifestyle methodologies that attempt to address toxic waste certainly improve 'health span' but none produce a meaningful extension in 'lifespan.'

## Adaptability is our greatest strength

I mean, what is it now; 4.5 million years out of Eastern Africa? We survived because we are apex omnivore predators. We are surprisingly good at surviving global catastrophic events [152,163] like droughts, glaciers and vulcanism because we can eat anything, unlike the specific diets of most animals. Our uniqueness to do this has produced a time-tested body, even durable enough to survive the insults thrown at the ecosystem by the sun. I would posit that modern man has lost ground in this fight but I think there is a way to return to this level of survivability.

We can adapt to just about any stress due to the very unusual and elastic characteristic of our genetics. We can eat anything because we had to adapt to rapid changes in food availability over vast stretches of time during environmental stress. Now our physical form can change to meet these challenges.

I think after millions of years of surviving these environmental stressors, homo sapiens have evolved to become a time-tested, protein dependent, regeneration machine that if maintained properly has no built in 'expiration date.

*Neogenesis*

# 3

# Human Phenotypic Plasticity

**Southeastern Africa about 4,000,000 years ago**
*"The lead Australopithecus female turned over one of the large, exposed anthracothere carcass leg bones from an earlier Hyaenodont kill baking in the hot afternoon sun and sniffed it. Something smelled good. She looked around, picked up a rock and hit the bone harder and harder until it broke open..."*

# Neogenesis

## Hmmm

Have you ever wondered how you can 'wonder' about an abstract idea like radical life extension? Or, in fact, any abstract idea? Even if most of humanity is not in awe of this capability, why do none of the other primates have this ability? It's our larger cerebral cortex, that the other primates never grew, that enables us to have this capability. And this unusual size is a result of our most valuable trait; to *physically change* to survive under extreme circumstances [1,2,3]. It's called phenotypic plasticity: the potential for morphological modifications, within genetically based constraints, in response to extended ecologically threatening conditions for a species survival. When its expressed magical things happen.

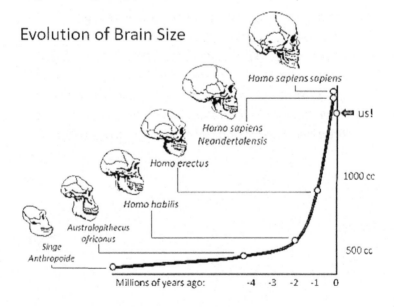

Evolution of Brain Size

Homo sapiens sapiens

⟸ us!

Homo sapiens
Neandertalensis

Homo erectus

1000 cc

Homo habilis

Australopithecus
africanus

Singe
Anthropoide

500 cc

Millions of years ago:  -4  -3  -2  -1  0

# Neogenesis

We grew our large brains during the 2.6 million yearlong Pleistocene global drought; a hard, nearly fatal, fight for survival that ended with the last solar micro nova 12,000 years ago. This late glacial period had large spreading polar ice encroaching on the only habitable regions of land. The land was unable to grow much vegetation because of the dryness from water vapor lifted high aloft at the equator and transported to the poles for ice accumulation. There was low $CO_2$ and variable temperatures; an environment hard to adapt to while competing with the herbivores also trying to survive (Richerson, Boyd, Bettinger; 2001).

Humans evolved alongside orangutans, chimpanzees, bonobos, and gorillas and all share a common ancestor from about 7 million years ago. But then, around 3.5 million years ago...Lucy appeared. We were plodding along for millions of years in the trees when the slow upward curve of the hominid brain size suddenly turns exponential around 2-4 million years ago. It looks as though we had figured something out.

## Something 'changed'

How did this ape start to exhibit an increasing brain size? It takes a lot of concentrated energy food to grow and operate a large brain. No other ape has exhibited the kinds of physical or psychological changes over the same time and no other ape has ever made a fire, cooked food, or made clothing.

We were certainly eating plant food that contained protein, but plants are lacking in several nutrients that help grow brains.

There has been a long debate about how we split off from the other primates and how we grew our larger brain-size, but the insight may have been glaringly evident all along...the fact that brains are mostly fat – 60 percent fat. What were the early hominids eating to get this ball rolling between four and six million years ago, to have the time for the appearance of Lucy? Plants?

No, they ate the plant eaters.

**Growing bigger brains requires calorie dense food**
Recently Dr. Jessica Thompson, at the Department of Anthropology at Emory University, has hypothesized that we didn't hunt and kill big animals at first for their meat [4]. We were too small, too slow, and too ill equipped to take down the megaherbivores the predators were taking for food. Rather we hunted for already killed large animals and scavenged their large bones [5]. Her hypothesis is that we were still developing our increasing brain size before its size and intellect allowed for making stone tools and flint knives. All of this developed in the humans because we were the first to hunt food for energy inside big bones and all we needed was a rock to break them open. Nutrient rich bone marrow is a concentrated source of vitamin B-12, riboflavin, iron, vitamin-E, thiamine, vitamin A and phosphorous and a 12 to 1 ratio of fat to protein (the

marrow is mostly fat) a nutrient-rich and hard to extract energy food protected by a hard bone that, when eaten, is concentrated in fat cells...like the brain. And all it took were rocks.

Rocks that later, much later, chipped flint into arrowheads.

**Some adjustments occurred along the way....**
We were becoming apex omnivore predators some 1,500,000 years ago. We were certainly eating meat with its fatty content to continue our brain development but maybe not cooked meat. It takes longer to digest raw meat [6].

Our appendix has been proposed to be an artifact from our distant past that helped us digest raw meat and the difficult to digest parts that came with it; nails, hair, bone bits, etc. [7]. The appendix still suppresses destructive antibodies by promoting immunity in the surrounding areas of the body and has an abundance of infection-fighting lymphoid cells. This suggests that it still plays a role in the immune system by producing and protecting good germs for the gut by 'rebooting' the digestive system [8,9]. The appendix might be another example of the pheno-plastic response; a result of stress long enough to stimulate a phenotypic-plastic response that 'made' a specific organ appear over millions of years due to the long-term nutrient stress of eating flesh.

# Neogenesis

*"Small opportunities can lead to great enterprises."*
-Demosthenes

**And then the Titan Prometheus gave us fire**
It took a while to produce 'Lucy,' but we were already on our way forward with fat, meat, and crude weapons. We were just awaiting...fire. And with fire we advanced to cooked food, even larger brains, then families, communities...oral and written history and ultimately knowledge over many lifetimes.

Fire...quite a game-changer, that one.

Our adoption of cooking food was pretty easy I imagine. It was easier to chew, it released a range of flavanol nutrients; and food tasted better cooked. This resulted in a huge change in our diet. Our brain was growing larger while we were eating uncooked meat but around 1,000,000 years ago, when we began eating cooked meat, we left the other primates far behind.

Instead of spending time spread out grazing in groups we spent more time gathered in groups around the fire staying warm and eating roasted meat and tubers together.

This 'social' change very likely gave us more opportunity to interact and improved communication with the members of the tribe advancing language, traditions, and customs; all of which may have helped hone our expanding brains to become even better problem solvers. It led us to our ability to record information with burnt sticks, charcoal and iron oxide

# Neogenesis

pigments on cave walls; left for future generations proving that long ago we made it to the level of intellect, not just survival.

> *"Eat diet food while you're waiting*
> *for the steak to cook."*
>
> *-Julia Childs*

Because of fire, the subsequent Homo variations were able to keep warm in the wildly varying climate and could spread far and wide. We may have stumbled upon this meat step during our evolution as scavengers, but it's the reason we have the big brain and why you can read this book.

Who would have thought? ...well, now you can.

## Our evolved genome

'It' (our genetic code) seems to have 'learned' to activate a pheno-plastic response to near-lethal or long-term stressors by reactively solving a problem by introducing new morphological physical changes to improve survival. This, I suspect, is a form of 'survival elasticity.' Our vestigial organs may be 'organ-medals'; artifacts from victorious battles fighting this war for millions of years...

But it's not about the battles...

## Being John Omnivore

Here's the reality: if you could be inside your head (and inside your cells) you would see you need nutrients and minerals from cooked and uncooked vegetable matter

35

and meat. Berries, nuts, fruit and other herbs, and plants as well those odd ones that we found by chance that helped evolve our ability to think in abstraction, the mind-altering plants and fungi. Some were essential for changing how our expanding brains processed thought and some of the 'psychedelic' experiences during this drug induced state was interpreted as 'spiritual' while 'under-the-influence' [10,11].

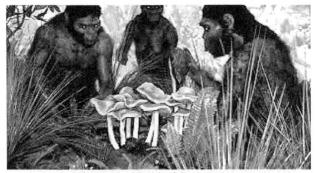

The Original Psychedelic Experience

These mysterious feelings have been used for thousands of years in hundreds of cultures ceremonially and religiously. They without question have expanded our 'idea' of consciousness.

In this light it's probably a good time to bring up the ELLI's; the outliers among us that may exhibit metabolic pheno-plastic modifications that give them a hedge against time; a genetic alteration to have a more active sirtuins and NAD+ profile.

ELLI's last into their 100's

# 4

# The ELLI Phenomena

*"God not only plays dice, but also sometimes throws them where they cannot be seen."*

-Dr. Stephen Hawking

## The outliers

Healthy aging is usually characterized by preserved cognitive and motor functions that decline as time passes. But there is a unique group of aging individuals, ELLI's, (exceptionally long lived individuals) that outlive the age of 100, with mostly intact cognition and physical health [12,13,14].

Two of the most-studied hallmarks of aging are DNA methylation and telomere attrition [15]. Normally epigenetic methylation and telomere shortening result in negative survival outcomes. Telomere shortening has long been documented to have inverse correlation with age, with mean telomere length (mTL) considered a marker for cellular senescence and aging [16,17,18,19,20,21,22]. The interesting result of testing ELLI's was the DNAmTL estimator found the telomere lengths of ELLI's to be approximately 500 bp 'shorter' than the control group.

That said, longer TL may have been associated with longevity through several potential mechanisms in the general population but not for ELLI's [23,24,25].

The other hallmark of aging, DNA methylation, increases with age. The DNA methylation of centenarians, however, seems to be 'slightly lower', hinting at a mechanism promoting healthy aging. Further, a study was performed on semi-supercentenarians (ages 105–109 years) and their offspring which demonstrated that both groups had younger 'epigenetic age' [26]. It was also found that offspring of the 105+ group age more slowly than that of age-matched controls and are 5.1 years younger. Overall, they averaged 8.6 years younger than the control group based on chronological age.

**Evidence of short time scale pheno-plastic modifications**

This ELLI phenomena may be a genetic modification because there is a ubiquitous, age-related decrease in global DNA methylation in this small population. It is not widespread throughout humanity and may be evidence of change on a relatively short timescale.

These tests infer that the reduction of methyl markers in the ELLI's is likely a unique genetic difference that produce higher levels of NAD+ that is passed to their offspring. It's known that methylation reduces access to histone and DNA codes for successful protein transcription – a critical aspect of cellular functionality and directly contributes to accelerated aging. It could also be said that they have more active SIRT6 which regulates aging, cancer, obesity, insulin resistance, inflammation, and energy metabolism.

Still, the more interesting finding is that the ELLI's had 'shorter' telomeres than the control group. This would suggest that telomere base numbers may be an indication of how many cell divisions have occurred but may not directly be equated with longevity. Rather, longevity is more related to the genetic integrity of the cells after division – e.g., lower methyl markers passed on during mitosis in daughter cells maintaining a younger functionality. This might contribute to the lower methylation test results in ELLI's. But sirtuins are only activated by NAD so this may be the insight to their longevity. NAD+ is essential for activating sirtuins, specifically SIRT1, SIRT6 and SIRT7 in the nucleus, that removes methyl and acetyl groups on histone and nuclear DNA to retain protein code pattern access. This ability to transcribe protein codes is also essential for preventing cellular senescence. This logically can be extrapolated to mean that higher levels of NAD+ correlate to longer lifespan by reducing the insults on genetic codes thereby allowing continued protein synthesis for functionality. And ELLI's seem to exhibit this enhanced capability. Critical depletion of NAD+ results in cell death through reduced ATP production and activation of apoptosis leading to a shorter lifespan [27].

Dry fasting – the non-eating metabolism – activates NAD+ synthesis and subsequently increases the sirtuins deacetylase activity (the removal of epigenetic markers). The metabolism of dry fasting has been shown to increase the NAD+/NADH ratio in cells (and mitochondria) to manufacture more NAD. This always results in the activation of the seven sirtuins, NAD+ dependent protein deacetylases, and lower methylation on code sequences [28,29]. L-tryptophan is the precursor (the molecular starting point) for synthesizing NAD, so you need to get it into your cellular factories by either eating foods that contain it or by consuming the amino acid as a supplement.

# Neogenesis

**Long lived species in nature**

These human examples are interesting but extremely long lifespans are rather common in the natural world. Bowhead whales are noted for long lifespans into the 210's, Koi live longer; some to 226. The Greenland shark is the oldest vertebrate on Earth that commonly live to 270 years but the oldest one recorded was nearly 400 (it could have been as old as 512). The ocean Quahog clam lives to over 500 years and then there are sponges. Sponges can live for thousands of years. Scientists have estimated two specimens to be 11,000 and 15,000 years old.

Zebra fish can turn on stem cells to even grow a new heart. Salamanders, Octopi, and frogs can re-grow limbs, lizard tails grow back when lost. These lifeforms exhibit genetic regeneration capability that must involve stem cells.

Lobsters and alligators have no cellular senescence and live until they succumb to attack, injuries that are too great to repair or simply getting stuck, but they do die eventually from old age.

And not surprisingly even immortality exists in nature. There are several species that never die.

Tardigrades are a phylum of water-dwelling, eight-legged, segmented micro-animals that can hyper hibernate. They can, after long spans of time, become biologically active in harsh environments, on space craft and even the near vacuum at the limits of our atmosphere. They are ubiquitous and may have hitched a ride to mars...where they might revive.

Turritopsis dohrnii is a species of jelly fish that can return into a small blob; it's first embryonic life stage. Muscle cells may become nerve cells, sperm, or eggs. Then, they can mature again and create hundreds of clones of itself. This happens if starving or injured. These common temperate ocean water creatures have been here since the beginning...they are immortal, they are still here.

Another is the simple hydra commonly found in freshwater lakes and ponds. Hydras are tiny (less than half an inch long) and last indefinitely by continually regenerating their cells. They show no signs of aging and most of their cells are stem cells...that must have activated telomerase...hydras can last indefinitely.

The common theme seen in these long-lived species is that they employ stem cells, a curious lack of senescence and or specific regeneration capabilities. And like The Phoenix Protocol, most of these species activate these life extension techniques during starvation and or stress.

Is there any reason to doubt that humans, who universally exhibit a rapid healing response to a wide spectrum of hormetic stressors, might also have a specific underlying capability to heal tissue and delay their expiration date?

# Neogenesis

I believe there is good evidence we do.

# So, What Are We?

*"Did you ever stop to think and forget to start"?*
-Winnie the Pooh

# 5

## I Think, Therefore I Am...I Think

*Each of us is experiencing a fully immersive experience in the moment of 'now' with only our 'self' at the center.*
*We never stop to think about 'how' we experience this and never ask... 'What' are we?*

# Neogenesis

We are four interlaced protein-based sensory bodies:

1) Bones
2) Organs, heart/vascular and brain/nervous system
3) Muscles
4) Fascial matrix

Molecularly the fascial matrix is an electromagnetic, nerve and biophoton signal conductive protein complex; not unlike an internal 'bio-intranet.' Only recently was it discovered that molecular interactions are organized by electro-magnetic fields; chemically activated by biophotons [30]. The body generates a stimulated emission of biophotons, light, by cells and mitochondria during molecular reactions. This was first reported by Fritz Albert Popp as 'energy spikes' in living tissue; stimulated photonic emission at specific frequencies that activate enzymatic reactions [31-34]. It has also been established those enzymatic cellular reactions release a cascade of biophotons which initiate subsequent reactions which then release more biophotons which initiates further reactions etc., etc.

Light is inducted, rejected, directed, and emitted by magnetic fields and indicates that the atomic bonds in molecules can be dramatically affected by light. Heat is infra-red light, but that discussion is beyond the scope of this book [169].

## Complete integration and interlacing

Protein structures within the matrix connect the skin, muscles and bones, through and to organs, and even create the extracellular matrix between cells that allows for information to find its way into the cells via their surface receptors [35,36,37,38,40]. The cell membrane surface pumps and receptors are the external connection to the complex architecture of cyto-plasm protein filaments: microtubules, actin, and intermediate filaments. These form an internal molecular highway and an internal scaffold to give cells shape. They also provide for the movement of mitochondria via 'walker proteins' that connect mitochondria to these microtubule highways. This highway enables them to go to 'a job site' to pump out ATP for ongoing intracellular metabolic processes where needed.

The cell membrane provides the 'network' connection receptors to open and allow entry into the cytoplasm. This process uses walker proteins to take a molecule once inside and 'walk' its chemical instructions down into the nucleus to stimulate protein synthesis for instance, or to lysosomes for degradation.

## A matrix with multi system functions

We are four interlaced and interlocked protein bodies that 'think'. Our multi system aspect may give us a measure of redundancy but our body would not work without a durable, resilient, structural architecture. Our body exists as a single continuous unit with a body-wide system of motion and motor pressure/stretch sensors permeating a web-like fascial matrix of collagen and glycoproteins that is always in a conversation with its brain.

This structural architecture has given us the ability to survive over millions of years. It allows us to sense the outside world in order to react and adjust the chemistry inside of our body in order to adapt to any challenge.

This is remarkable in and of itself, but it clearly displays our unusually reactive genetic plasticity that has contributed to our long list of metabolic survival capabilities associated with maintaining and regenerating these four interlaced protein dependent systems.

**The fascial matrix is mostly collagen** Your body has more collagen and elastin in its skin, bones, muscles, and the fascial inner-web matrix than any other protein. Collagen and elastin provide the tensegrity, a structural principle using compressed components (which do not touch each other – bone) inside a network of protein 'cables' (tendons attached to muscle and bone) providing continuous tension to give our body elasticity and resilience. Stretch and 'spring-back' [42].

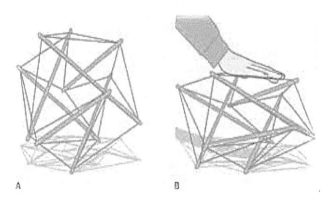

A                    B

Collagen helps preserve the elasticity in skin, and it is the primary building block for nails, hair, teeth, and bones. One of the main health benefits of collagen is its powerful anti-inflammatory properties, important in the prevention of diseases such as arthritis. Collagen, like DNA, needs to be adequately hydrated to perform its function.

**Fascial trains**
There is also a pervasive fascial band system; long ligament sheeting beneath the skin that is interlaced into the proteins of the connective tissue below it [37]. This matrix system gives our body its unique and amazing elastic range of motion.

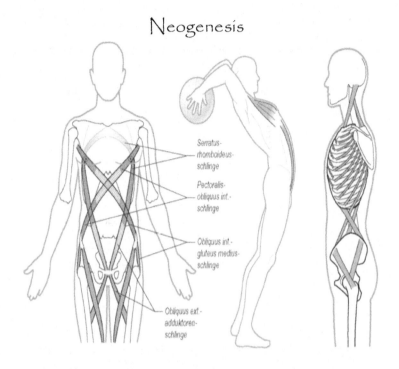

## Coordination of all parts

The entire facial matrix is also loaded with unique motion, stretch and pressure sensory cells within the fascia that transmit to nerves and to the brain for evaluating the environment [43].

The interstitial sensors are high- and low-pressure signal sensors found everywhere even inside bones with the highest concentration in the periosteum; the thick membrane that surrounds the length of bones.

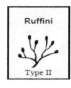

The Ruffini sensors are lateral stress and sustained pressure sensors found in ligaments of peripheral joints, dura matter, and tissue utilized for stretching.

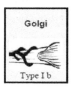

The Golgi sensors are stretch sensors that wrap around the tendons connected to organs to regulate contraction, joint stretch sensors, ligaments of peripheral joints.

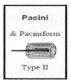

The Pacini sensors are for rapid pressure changes and vibration found at the muscle and tendon cell interface and spinal ligaments. These are found as relatively thin fibrous membranes which sheath layers of muscle.

One of the most unusual findings of studying the facial matrix is that a deep tissue massage is not as effective at relieving tension in this system as simple superficial stimulation (Swedish massage). A light touch has been shown to relieve the bound-up collagen fibrins; letting them unwind and relax. This in turn sometimes takes tension off areas expressing 'phantom pain' by relaxing locked strands of the matrix pulling on those same areas that 'hurt'. It is thought that the gentle touch works by providing a more beneficial, calm, and non-threatening stimuli.

**Everything is interlaced to react to stress**
The muscle and bone system stresses (anabolic load and anabolic impact stress) are triggers to affect

positive cellular, muscular, neural and organ performance. The condition of teeth affects major organs and body function. Seen under electron microscopy we are a genetically coded structurally interwoven quasi-system of bones, organs and muscles all held inside a mesh-like matrix of specialized, organ-specific collagen and proteoglycans – (hyaluronic acid 'springs').

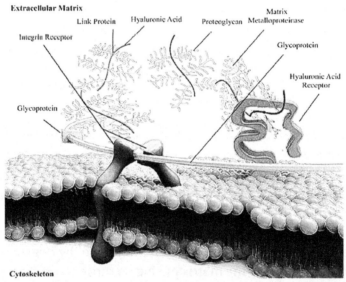

It exists between cells and inside the protein membranes and compartments holding everything together in shape and in their place. To get a sense of how pervasive and comprehensive this protein matrix is, consider some of the different connective tissue types providing this flexible system of shape-memory like protein structures:

- Mechanical fibrillar collagens and elastin provide tensile strength, recoil, and tissue shape memory.
- Proteoglycans act as 'structured water' storage in the intercellular matrix and provide cushioning.
- Small leucine-rich repeat proteins that assemble the fascial matrix fibers and cartilage.
- Glycoproteins that bind cells along these microscopic highways.

In other words, it has billions of channels of spiraling collagen that not only hold things in a 'spring-y' resilient protein web, it also conducts electric impulses, photons and chemical signals like a wiring harness to cells and organs.

### The fascial matrix repair crew

The matrix is maintained by cells called fibroblasts; normally these are slow metabolizing, sleepy cells that crawl around inside the extra cellular matrix and repair about 2% of the matrix per month. That's how durable it is. However, if there is hypertension, crisis, or injury they 'pheno-convert' by chemical triggers. They then stop moving around and 'tent' down and start putting out a lot of proteins fibers, this can lead to fibrosis.

### The fascial primo vascular system

The outer layer of the fascia, the skin, is porous. Water is channeled through skin, via a twelve meridian tension line system of micro fibrin vessels. This allows for the skin to conduct water deeply into the body to hydrate the muscles, organs, and bones. This is probably why an Epsom salt bath and swimming in the ocean feels so good.

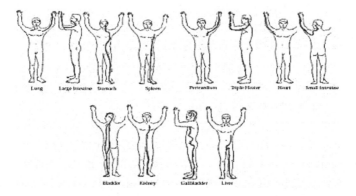

Lung　Large Intestine　Stomach　Spleen　Pericardium　Triple Heater　Heart　Small Intestine

Bladder　Kidney　Gallbladder　Liver

This is a deep reservoir of emergency water, like a camel's stomach. It's an organized fluid system within the fascial system that corresponds to the ancient acupuncture meridians.

Expanding on the earlier work of Professor B.H. Kim, who first described it, Prof. K.S. Soh and his team at the Seoul National University has developed methods to detect and identify this new anatomical fluid system [44,45,46]. He named it the primo vascular system (PVS), and they renamed the channels and nodes within the system as primo vessels (PV) and primo nodes (PN).

# Neogenesis

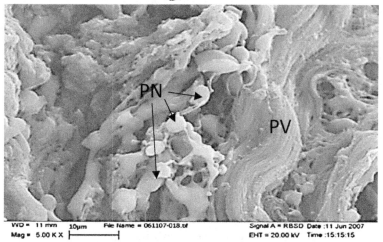

The Primo System: Organized collagen networks for systems distribution

The name 'primo' is well chosen because these vessels are primordial vessels that develop during embryogenesis, before the blood and the nervous system form as the foundation architecture for their development. The PVS is an independent functional morphological system. This system provides the original conduits for vascular, lymphatic vessels and nerves.

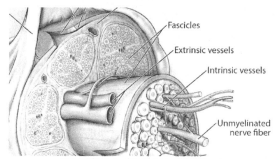

Coinciding mulit-systems architecture

# Neogenesis

The PVS also contains hormones and microcells with chromosomes. Thus, the particularities of different body systems are combined in the PVS. The superficial PVs and extravascular PVs are connected to superficial nodes. The deep PVs are connected between them with intravascular PVs, deep PNs and organ nodes. During dry fasting the PVS assists the repair and regeneration of cells and tissues.

## System architecture
The diameters of the lumens of a PV are only 5–10 μm, which is of capillary size like the blood and lymphatic systems. The biochemical components of primo fluids are nucleic and ribonucleic acids, nitrogen, fats, reducing sugar, hyaluronic acid, 19 free amino acids, and 16 free mononucleotides. The PVS carries the basic substances to create proteins. It is proposed that it supplies cells and tissues with substances for recovery and regeneration of damaged structures. The primo fluid helps damaged cells recover their structures by constructing new proteins. The DNA in the PVS fluid carries information on how to repair the cells. Hyaluronic acid is a glycosaminoglycan distributed widely throughout connective, epithelial, and neural tissues. It is formed in the plasma membrane instead of the Golgi apparatus in the cell and contributes significantly to cell proliferation and migration.

## In the beginning
The duplication of the PVS by the vascular and the nervous systems begins with the creation of the

primordial PVS in the very earliest stage of embryonic development. In fact, the primordial PVS provides the vascular and the nervous systems the architecture to form around the PVS. In this case, the PVS combines the features of the vascular, the nervous, and the hormonal systems. It's how osteocalcin, once released by exercise, moves from the periosteum into the system.

Subsequently, after all embryonic body systems have developed, the primordial PVS remains connected with them, but dominates and controls them as the oldest morphological functional system.

Hematopoietic organs such as bone marrow, the spleen, and lymphatic nodes, are probably the largest source of the microcells that go into the primo fluid in the well-developed network of the PVs and distributed to the target organs. Living organisms keep themselves alive via regeneration following the sanal-cell cycle. Sanals (microcells) grow into cells, and cells in turn become the sanals. A sanalsome is a kind of chromosome that forms when cells divide.

The microcells have the characteristics of embryonic stem cells, which is probably why they participate in the regeneration of cells and tissues.

**Amino acid intake is the key to Neogenesis**
Amino acids are not only required for making collagen; they are also essential for multiple cellular and biochemical functions. They are the means for maintaining our four body interlaced systems.

**Tryptophan** helps in the formation of serotonin and melatonin. It's the precursor molecule for NAD synthesis; essential for demethylation.

**Threonine** is involved in the formation of vitamin B12, it intervenes in the regeneration of collagen proteins and helps the body to recover from wounds at the muscle level.

**Isoleucine** is important for protein development and for energy storage, necessary for the synthesis of hemoglobin and helps the body to recover after intense physical activity.

**Leucine** activates mTOR, it's critically important for the formation and maintenance of muscle tissue, skin, and bones.

**Lysine** is needed to create L-carnitine, it allows the circulation of oxygen in muscle tissues and is involved in the metabolism of lipids.

**Methionine** is involved in metabolism and helps to burn fat; it's needed for the formation of other amino acids and for reducing muscle degeneration and fat in the liver as well as keeping skin and nails healthy.

And that's just six of the twenty.

**Sanity and mood are dependent on amino acids**
There's a long list of conditions from the dysfunction resulting from a deficiency in the production of the neurotransmitter serotonin. Food cravings, negativity, depression, worry, anxiety, low self-esteem, obsessive thoughts or behaviors, controlling, perfectionism,

winter blues, irritability, rage (PMS), dislike hot weather, panic attacks or phobias, fibromyalgia, jaw pain, suicidal thoughts, night owl, hard to sleep, insomnia, disturbed sleep.

The body will seek sweets, starch, tobacco, chocolate, ecstasy, marijuana, alcohol for their endorphin stimulating effects to seek relief from the emotional aspect of this type of dysfunction. Many of these 'food solutions' contain L-tryptophan. L-tryptophan is an essential amino acid that cannot be synthesized by humans, although some is manufactured by gut bacteria. It is however usually scavenged by the macrophages that employ it to biochemically attack and neutralize invaders. So together, the immune system and endocrine system demands alone can create low levels leading to dysfunction.

Tryptophan is essential for synthesis of both serotonin and melatonin. Tryptophan is methylated to create serotonin which is then acetylated to create melatonin in the pineal gland. Without L-tryptophan to prevent deficiency, things can go haywire.

You know the drill: get more in your diet by pill, banana, turkey, all the usual suspects to keep on an 'even keel.'

Another one is tyrosine (in one form or another).

### Happiness and alertness

Catecholamines are hormones that the brain, nerve tissues, and adrenal glands produce that are derived from the amino acid tyrosine.

# Neogenesis

Catecholamines are the really big ones for being 'on the ball', alertness. Adrenaline, noradrenaline, and dopamine are physiologically important neurotransmitters as part of the sympathetic and central nervous systems. If your body lacks tyrosine, several systems don't or can't work.

This group of chemicals are needed to interact with adrenergic receptors inside the facial matrix to produce a sharp state of alertness. The body releases catecholamines in response to emotional or physical stress but depletes tyrosine to produce the response. Not knowing how to address the deficiency, our ancient mind deliberately produces solutions in the form of cravings. Sugar, starch, tobacco, weed, cocaine, pills, and foods that contain tyramine derived from tyrosine that acts as a catecholamine releasing agent. It's one reason I eat canned sardines. Canned sardines have almost a gram, .08-gm of tyramine per 100 grams as well as 3 grams of omega-3.

The take away from this section is that all the fascial system is made of collagen and is another reason it is so important to eat protein for the building blocks that make collagen.

Neogenesis

# 6

# Longer If You're Stronger

*"If you don't use it, you lose it"*

# Neogenesis

## Sarcopenia and osteoporosis

Sarcopenia is the loss of muscle, strength, and function and one of the most pervasive health problems in the elderly, while osteoporosis is the most common bone disease where bones become weak and brittle [153,154]. The truth is, older people don't fall over and break their hip, their hip breaks, then they fall over.

Ultimately both conditions lead to frailty which is the leading cause of death in older people and sadly neither of these conditions are recognized as treatable.

I think both are a result of 'user error' and both are preventable and treatable.

Sarcopenia results from not eating at least a minimal amount of protein to provide an adequate level of the amino acid leucine to make muscle cells. Osteoporosis is caused by the reduction of the bone hormone, osteocalcin needed for bone formation and only released during exercise.

Sarcopenia and osteoporosis have nothing to do with chronological age. It happens over time by whatever means, financial, sociological, or psychological by eating below the minimum level of protein sources daily and not exercising.

Protein (amino acids) and exercise build muscle and, when combined, always improves bone density. Like 'old blue eyes' said: *"you can't have one without the other."*

# Neogenesis

Bone health is essential for an extended lifespan. Bone marrow produces the immune system cells and bone releases the osteocalcin necessary for a long list of related body system functionality but there's more to the picture.

Exercise is the greatest physiological stress that our bodies normally experience and because it takes some effort, hardly anyone does it.

*"To get back my youth I would do anything in the world, except take exercise, get up early, or be respectable."*
*-Oscar Wilde – The Picture of Dorian Gray*

It's a common theme.

This is glaringly obvious by the increasing number of elderly people in nursing homes today who suffer from this epidemic of frailty. If you don't exercise to maintain your skeletomuscular system, this is an inevitability. Today, it's the rule not the exception that you will end up in a nursing home if you don't do everything in your power to prevent it. You literally don't have any time to 'waste'.

Exercise is dose dependent so embrace it.

Given the physiological stress associated with exercise and the adaptations that occur to handle this stress (vascular elasticity and durability), it is not surprising that exercise is known to prevent or effectively treat a multitude of degenerative conditions including cardiovascular disease, cancer, diabetes, depression,

Alzheimer's disease, Parkinson's disease, and many others [168].

**Making muscle begins inside cells**
mTOR (mammalian mechanistic target of rapamycin) forms two multiprotein complexes, mTORC1 and mTORC2 and are composed of discrete protein binding partners to regulate cell growth, motility, and metabolism. mTORC1 and mTORC2 regulate each other. These complexes are sensitive to distinct stimuli: mTORC1 is sensitive to nutrient stimulation. mTORC2 is responsive to growth factor signaling. What most researchers don't explain is that mTOR (C1 & C2) integrate nutrient and mitogen signals to regulate cell growth to increase cell mass and cell size as well as activating cell division. 'Muscle turnover' is a fancy term that many fail to explain. Muscle turnover is the replacement of old muscle cells with new ones by mitosis that occurs after activating the mTOR complex [26].

**Exercise and mTOR**
Many of the health benefits of exercise are mediated by mTOR not only within the working muscle, but also in not-so distant tissues such as fat, liver, and brain. Of course, this makes sense since these organs and systems are found along-side most muscles in the body. Exercise activates mTOR in diverse tissues and is important, from this adaptive response to exercise, because it keeps us bigger, stronger, longer lasting, and healthier as a result [47]. mTOR complex is only

activated when all the parts are present: growth factors, nutrients, and amino acids. Amino acids are essential to maintain both muscle and bone to have a durable, resilient body that can easily cope with the stresses of an extended lifespan. And that's where exercise comes in because exercise stimulates bone to produce a hormone critical to all of this.

## Osteocalcin

Bones are an endocrine organ that secretes a variety of important hormones. Osteocalcin is a very important hormone produced by the bones during impact or load stress - exercise.

Osteocalcin helps lock calcium into bones in its active form and increase their strength and healing. Studies suggest that once released into the blood, it helps adjust insulin and blood sugar levels, increases testosterone, muscle mass and muscle strength, and even improves brain function.

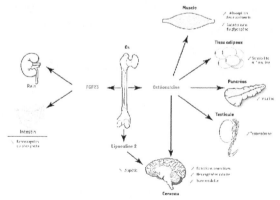

Osteocalcin – A hormone with a wide range of actions

# Neogenesis

Impact and load stress are types of anabolic stress triggers to signal bone growth. Exercise is necessary to stimulate production of osteocalcin. Bone marrow and the periosteum (reactive to load and impact stress) is loaded with it. And it's the periosteum, a fascia matrix protein structure, that produces stem cells necessary for this activity.

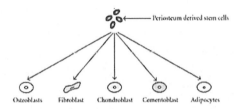

Different cells types derived from Periosteum

Osteocalcin is released into the blood during impact or stress exercise (jumping rope, sprinting, rebounding, weight resistance training). When osteocalcin is released it:

- increases the production of insulin by the pancreas and adjusts blood glucose levels [63, 64]
- stimulates testosterone production [65]
- increases muscle strength [66]
- improves brain function [63]

## Osteocalcin helps reverse osteoporosis

Osteoporosis occurs when bone strength deteriorates due to decreases in bone mineral content (BMC) and bone mineral density (BMD), the most basic markers of bone metabolism, as well as changes in bone microarchitecture; all of which occur with aging [67]. Only recently has it been discovered that levels of the bone hormone osteocalcin, responsible for binding calcium to bones, is released during physical exertion. It's presence in the blood stream determines whether your skeleton will erode or not. For this process of calcium deposition and bone strength to occur, osteocalcin first needs to be activated by vitamin K2 [68].

**Explaining the far-reaching effects of exercise**
In the pancreas, osteocalcin increases insulin production. It also increases the number of beta cells that produce, store, and release insulin [69,70]. In addition, osteocalcin acts on muscles and other tissues by keeping sugar levels in check. It works by increasing the production of adiponectin in fat cells (adipocytes). Adiponectin, in turn, increases the uptake of glucose into fat and muscle cells [71,72]. Low levels of osteocalcin can impair the body's ability to use insulin to control glucose levels [73,74].

Osteocalcin increases the production of testosterone in testes for more growth hormone during exercise [75,76,65,77,78].

Osteocalcin may increase the strength of skeletal muscles indirectly. It helps the muscles adapt to exercise, which is particularly important for preventing sarcopenia in older people [79,80,66,81,82]. Strong muscles work to make strong bones.

# Neogenesis

Higher levels of blood osteocalcin have been linked to muscle strength in women over the age of 70. Plus, adequate osteocalcin levels reduce the risk of falls and bone fractures by maintaining muscle mass.

## Multiple systems require osteocalcin

Several studies suggest that osteocalcin levels affect brain health and may be able to enhance cognitive function by increasing key neurotransmitters dopamine, noradrenaline, and serotonin. In one study of women between the ages of 71 and 78 years, higher osteocalcin levels were associated with better cognitive function [84].

Conversely, low osteocalcin levels were linked to negative changes in the microstructure of the brain (the corpus striatum in the cerebrum of the brain, hypothalamus, thalamus, putamen, and subcortical white matter) and subsequently reduces cognitive performance since the corpus striatum is where reward and control, behavior and sleep control, cognitive and motor function is managed [83].

## High and low osteocalcin levels

Low osteocalcin blood levels have been associated with type 2 diabetes in men, women, and children [85,86,87,88, 89,90]. In turn, high osteocalcin was associated with better control of blood glucose levels in a study of 128 people with type 1 diabetes [91]. But it's still not clear whether it is osteocalcin that affects glucose levels or the other way around [92].

Interestingly, osteocalcin levels and stiffness in the arteries were related in an "inverted J-shaped curve." This means that both low and high levels of osteocalcin may increase the risk of hardening of the arteries, although low levels likely increase the risk to a greater degree [93]. Low levels of osteocalcin have been associated with heart disease.

## Osteocalcin and metabolic syndrome

Metabolic syndrome is a cluster of the following conditions that together increase a person's risk of heart disease and diabetes:

- high blood pressure
- high blood sugar
- excess body fat around the waist
- abnormal cholesterol levels
- high triglyceride levels

In a meta-analysis of 55 studies with 47k people, low osteocalcin blood levels were associated with metabolic syndrome. Similarly, in 798 older men, low levels pointed to metabolic syndrome [94,94]. Additionally, in a study of over 2,000 people, lower osteocalcin levels were associated with higher levels of C-reactive protein (CRP), a marker of chronic inflammation in people with metabolic syndrome [95]. According to a meta-analysis of 28 studies with a total of over 18.6k participants, people with low osteocalcin levels were more likely to have a higher body mass index (BMI). Studies in children, adolescents, and pre- and post-menopausal women support this association [96,97, 98,99,100,101].

# Neogenesis

In a non-alcoholic fatty liver syndrome study of 120 children aged 7 to 13 years old (60 NAFLD patients and 60 controls), low osteocalcin blood levels predicted the severity of NAFLD. Low levels were also an indicator of NAFLD in four studies that included almost 9k adults [102,103,104,105,106]. Animal studies suggest that osteocalcin improves NAFLD by activating the Nrf2 protein (the master regulator of antioxidant and detox enzymes), which reduces oxidative stress [107].

## Exercise is the trigger

Serum levels of osteocalcin (formation of new bone marker) and deoxypyridinoline (DPD) (break down of old bone marker) are used to determine the effects of exercise on bone formation. (Woitge et. al. 1998) conducted a comparative study of aerobic exercise and resistance exercise in relation to bone metabolism. In the aerobic exercise, the osteocalcin level decreased on the fourth week and then recovered on the eighth week while (DPD) continued to decrease indicating reduced remineralization over time. In the resistant exercise the levels of osteocalcin and DPD increased for both four weeks and eight weeks. The researchers concluded that while aerobic training led to changes compatible with reduced bone resorption activity, resistance training results in an overall accelerated bone turnover. Therefore, the impact of physical activity on bone turnover specifically depends on the kind of exercise performed.

# Neogenesis

## Rebounding

As mentioned earlier, rebounding (jumping on a mini trampoline) is one of the best exercises to release osteocalcin. Rebounding is used by NASA to regrow both bone and muscle in astronauts after being in zero gravity during on-orbit missions. Bone and muscle are made to counter gravity and shrink in size in zero-G [108]. Rebounding raises heart rate, oxygen uptake is increased, and, in fact, the magnitude of the biomechanical stimuli is greater than with running. It supplies the impact stress necessary to stimulate osteocalcin release with every bounce. Your body can experience up to 4Gs of gravitational force without any joint shock and flex 75 trillion cells 100 times per minute in a 10-minute session.

The increased G force on the bones strengthens them with less risk of injury than other forms of exercise. The loading and unloading of muscles also increase strength yet the gravitational forces are evenly distributed throughout the body minimizing injury or potential rupture of muscles, ligaments, or tendons. Rebounding's effectiveness for strengthening bone density can help stop osteoporosis and even reverse the damage. The bouncing motion also helps the lymphatic system.

So, yeah, it's not a joke; run for your life or even better...
bounce for your life.

# Neogenesis

# 7

# The 3-Minute Workout

*"Muscle is the longevity organ."*
-Dr. Gabrielle Lyons

*"Heavy Duty training is basically a strength training
program but in order to get bigger
you've got to get stronger."*
-Mike Mentzer

# Neogenesis

**The 3-Minute Workout**

I can only tell you what I did to get *stronger* and *build muscle and bone* at 69 years old. This consisted of a 3-minute workout focusing on a rotating cycle of working a different body part each day; chest, shoulders, back, legs, glutes, arms (biceps & triceps) and exerting as much effort as I could for 3 minutes using a high intensity strength training method. Sometimes daily, sometimes skip a day but a regular routine most of the time. It's supposed to be impossible to build strength and muscle at my age; 69 years old. But this technique produced remarkable results and I increased my strength and muscle mass in a very short amount of time. For example, I started with 90 pounds on the leg press machine, and in no time at all I was able to leg press 540 pounds.

**How long is this workout?**

Three minutes is the actual amount of time you spend 'lifting the weight' and not necessarily the amount of time you spend in the gym; it's only a commitment of 21 minutes per week if you work out daily.

High-intensity training, commonly known as Heavy Duty, HIT or peak output, is a form of strength training popularized in the 1970s by Arthur Jones, the founder of Nautilus. The training focuses on performing quality weight training repetitions to the point of momentary muscular failure. You must perform the exercises correctly and be conscious of your form. Additionally, it may help to have a training partner who can spot you when need be.

# Neogenesis

I'm promoting this method for Neogenesis for one reason; it's the fastest way to grow muscle and bone to prevent sarcopenia and osteoporosis, the two conditions that assure you will not last. This program reverses the bone loss that leads to disability and frailty and frailty is the leading cause of death in the elderly.

**Background**

The 3-minute workout is based on the earlier work of Durk Pearson and Sandy Shaw from their book, *The Life Extension Weight Loss Program* (1986) pg.31, 'Sandys Lucky Break'. In the spring of 1979 Sandy broke her foot. Coincidently, this happened at the same time she and Durk were experimenting with nutrients that employed the amino acid arginine to stimulate growth hormone for building muscle and losing fat. So, she decided to take this GH releasing nutrient while performing an upper body only workout program [since she couldn't use her foot].

Sandy took 10 grams of the GH releasing nutrient on an empty stomach 1 hour before performing a daily total of 2 to 3 minutes of 'peak output' bench press and bicep curls. At 6 weeks of using the supplement and 2 to 3 minutes of intense, training to failure exercise per day, Sandy put on about 5 pounds of muscle, lost 25 pounds of fat and her foot healed in half the time the doctors said it would heal. She hadn't reduced her caloric intake either.

They later developed a product called *Inner Power* based on their earlier arginine supplement that produced these remarkable results, rapid strength and muscle growth, rapid healing.

Because of the success of their experiment, I decided to try their method.

The Neogenesis 3-minute workout incorporates Durk and Sandys' earlier work using their arginine supplement taken one hour before a workout to allow time for it to get into the blood stream and get to the brain to stimulate the pituitary gland to release growth hormone. Arginine supplementation is known to stimulate nitric oxide release by endothelial cells to relax blood vessels, and thereby helping to provide more blood, insulin, amino acids, and available growth hormones to the muscle cells during exercise. Timing is everything.

The arginine supplement that I take one hour before working out is *Inner Power* designed by Life Enhancement (*see page 144*).

I added a second supplement my routine; *Perfect Amino*, which I generally take after my workout (*see page 144*). The amino acid supplement makes sure I get amino acids right after the workout instead of eating protein. Protein takes time to digest back into amino acids and instead of making the muscles wait for amino acids, the amino complex immediately provides the ingredients to start repair. A half hour later I eat or drink protein.

## It's all in the details

Forty years later we now know that l-arginine does not directly stimulate GH, but rather suppresses a GH suppressor, somatostatin. Somatostatin suppresses GH-releasing hormone so the GH producing cells don't get the signal to release GH [108,132]. By blocking the inhibitor, more GH is available. The benefits of improving growth hormone levels are diverse, including increasing the use of fat as a fuel as well as insulin and insulin-growth factor-1 (IGF-1) levels.

Additionally, the effects of exercise are amplified by osteocalcin 'the bone hormone'; which is released during the workout and increases testosterone levels; further increasing growth hormone levels [66,79].

The 3-minute workout is a great way to adopt a regular exercise habit. You can always alter the program, and you probably will as you progress, but this is a good starting point. I was 69 years old when I started and had never worked out or lifted weight heavier than a surfboard.

After seeing the benefits of this program, I will always work out.

# Neogenesis

**Here's my routine on days I work out.**

**8:00 AM**
Up drinking my morning coffee.

**10:00 AM**
I take 12 grams of Inner Power (on and empty stomach) one hour before working out. The arginine supplement starts nitric oxide stimulation of the vascular wall and suppresses somatostatin to improve growth hormone levels.

**11:00 AM**
When I get to the gym I do an intense work-out to failure routine exactly one hour after taking the arginine supplement. I lift as heavy a weight as I can until I can't...that's lift to failure. The total time lifting is only 3 minutes. When I can safely perform 10 reps of a set, I increase the weight. After my workout I eat a banana to replenish the glycogen levels in my muscles and a half teaspoon Redmond Sea Salt to replenish salt loss [170].

**After the workout: 50 grams of protein**
I take 5 to 10 Perfect Amino tablets with a large glass of water and wait 30 minutes before having a protein drink, tuna salad or a couple of tins of sardines / anchovies.

**Dinner: 50 grams of protein**
I eat a good lean protein along with vegetables or green salad for dinner...see the theme here? I try to eat food that provides leucine and micronutrient mineral elements. These foods don't spike insulin before I go to sleep, and I stop eating at least 3 hours before hitting the sack.

# Neogenesis

## Sleep

And get a good night's sleep. Muscles grow when you rest, exercise is just a trigger to activate the mechanisms for muscle cellular synthesis. It only makes sense that when the body is asleep and muscles aren't being used that growth occurs.

## The reason growth hormone decreases with age

A decreasing number and size of growth hormone (GH) producing cells in the pituitary may be the reason growth hormone is reduced as we age. Testing in aged mice has shown that both Growth Hormone Releasing-Hormone (GHRH) producing cells, (*the one that instruct the GH cells to release GH*) and the somatostatin producing cells (SS) are fewer as expected, by age and attrition, but there's a puzzle: the ratio of the number of SS cells in old mice is greater than the number of GHRH cells.

It is thought that the fall in the number and size of GH cells in the pituitary gland, with age, may be related to the recorded increase in the ratio of the number of SS cells in the hypothalamus over time; the suppressor of GHRH [133]. Can we reset that balance?

## Dry fasting to the rescue

Maybe we do have the ability to restore growth hormone releasing cells. In recent mice studies, the pituitary gland has demonstrated that although cell turnover is normally low, pituitary stem cells do exist and can regenerate pituitary endocrine cell types in response to physiological stressors such as starvation

# Neogenesis

[115,136]. Additional evidence for the presence of pituitary stem cells comes from studies showing that SOX2+ pituitary cells, from embryos and adults, can differentiate into multiple pituitary endocrine cell types in vitro and in vivo, suggesting that these cells are multipotent (109,110,112,113,114).

During day 3 of a 7-day dry fast, the regeneration activation of stem cells in all the stem cell niches may regenerate the tissue in the pituitary and hypothalamus stem cell niches as well. This may act to restore the size and number of the GHRH cells and may reset the balance with SS cells to establish a new, higher level of GH output. This may be why I am seeing substantial muscle growth at age 69 after my third 7-day dry fast.

Perhaps, over time, the endocrine system cells in the pituitary can be restored during the dry fasting cycles to return growth hormone levels to a younger concentration as tissue is remodeled with young stem cell replacements.

Time will tell.

# 8

# Inflammation is the Slow Death

*Inflamm-aging' is a chronic, low-grade inflammation, that develops with advanced age and leads to immunosenescence. Inflamm-aging is intensively associated with many aging diseases.*

# Neogenesis

## A metabolic albatross

The main theme of my theory of normal aging is that our bodies wear out because the accumulation of some of the more damaging metabolic garbage (created during the daily eating metabolism) reaches a threshold. Death in this scenario is by user error. By increasing the fuel for cellular fires by eating without ever cleaning the cellular environment, a chronic, low-level inflammation is created. This kind of background inflammation is an ever increasing 'drag on the system' that will reliably cause a critical sub system to fail that the rest rely on. Normal 'aging' is in large part from unprotected cellular function insults causing an erosion of function. The insults are usually prevented by a robust army of different immune system cells. But an aging immune system is like any army that, at one point, faces over whelming odds as it slowly runs out of ammo; it leads only to reduction in force where what's left are zombies - senescent immune system cells.

A state of immunosenescence.

## Cells on fire make tissue on fire

Our cells are like the houses in a city. Our immune system is exactly like the fire department. The trash that accumulates in and around our cells can catch fire - inflame if you will. These metabolic fires are put out rather efficiently during our youth. I'm sure you've noticed this as 'youthfulness.' But the house fires that may be extinguished in our youth grow in number because the fuel, the metabolic trash, accumulates as time goes on from the daily eating metabolism.

The number of house fires grow over time until the fire department is unable to put them all out or must to move on to a new, more urgent fire, leaving some to smolder. But as the city ages, the fire department equipment gets broken, hoses get holes, fire fighters are lost and it's only a matter of time before the whole city catches fire and burns down. This is normal human aging because the body or the city, in this example, never removes the growing metabolic trash that is constantly catching fire. The smoldering fires are the hallmarks of [inflame]-aging.

## The hallmarks of aging

These hallmarks are due to the ever-increasing trash and omega-6 oil damage to mitochondria (from specific vegetable and seed oils) and a long list of bad chemicals from the biosphere that causes mitochondrial dysfunction (*an ever reducing energy production*), altered metabolic signaling (*sending the wrong signal to get the job done*), defective autophagy and mitophagy (*cells organelles aren't repaired*), dysbiosis (*gut bacteria imbalance*), diminished proteostasis (*the ability to manufacture needed proteins in cells*), stem cell exhaustion (*genetic code tagging leading to the inability to replicate*), telomere attrition (*erosion of the ends of the chromosomes leading to zombie cells*), epigenetic changes (*loss of protein code access*), genomic instability (*unrepaired genetic breaks, damage and lost* code), and cellular and immune system senescence (*a state where cells no longer work to provide life force*) [48,49,50].

An impairment of any of these hallmarks can promote inflammation and affect the other hallmarks [50]. The causal driver of inflammation is an accumulation of damaged cells, cell debris, and misfolded molecules that accumulate during the eating metabolism and can't be deconstructed in a night's sleep. These hallmarks are interconnected and co-occur with one another, but all converge on chronic inflammation.


## The Cells That Fight Inflammation

### Macrophages are your fire fighters

Macrophages are phagocytes; cells that are supposed to protect the body by ingesting harmful foreign particles, toxins, bacteria, and dead or dying cells. These are special immune system cells that are mobile, moving into and out of tissue to fix problems.

Macrophages play a critical role in keeping the body working correctly and regulating inflammation. It's an evolved automatic response to the causal drivers of inflammation, chemically sensed by pattern recognition receptors to activate macrophage cells to address the problems. But as the toxic debris builds up in the bone marrow, where they are created, they too undergo changes that ultimately contribute to the age-related pathologies as they become damaged, contributing to inflammation. Macrophages are central in this phenomenon [116]. And there are two types of macrophages: M1 and M2.

## M1 / pro-inflammatory
M1 act to break matter down (catabolic) and because of this are bactericidal. They are normally glycolytic; converting glucose into pyruvate to enter the pathway to make ATP. M1 macrophages also secrete a variety of inflammatory and bactericidal mediators; all of which increase in circulation with age as the debris they are designed to remove also increases with age [117,118].

## M2 / anti-inflammatory
M2 are involved in tissue repair, angiogenesis, and phagocytosis [119, 120]. They represent the opposite end of the polarization spectrum from M1 macrophages. They rely mainly on oxidative phosphorylation and fatty acid oxidation for energy and are turned on during dry fasting.                    But under the chronically challenging conditions caused by the accumulation of metabolic garbage, the 'normal' switch to the M2 phenotype is impaired.

## Eating and non-eating affects the switch
Macrophages react to chemical switches during eating and nightly sleep to differentiate into their pro-inflammatory or anti-inflammatory roles. Over time the chemical switches can be affected by the increasing amount of cellular toxins and debris and become confused as to which one to differentiate into.

# Neogenesis

Non-eating periods lead to a phenotypic switch from the M1 to the M2 anti-inflammatory type. Not surprisingly, the switch to M2 is during the period of non-eating. But because the local microenvironment is becoming ever more toxic by not enacting a dry fasting cleaning cycle, the accumulation of this cellular garbage plays a critical role in shaping what genes are expressed in the cells that the macrophages are trying to maintain [121].

In this toxic environment, incorrect biochemical signals take place and macrophages can display both M1 and M2 markers. No longer exclusively pro-inflammatory or anti-inflammatory [119].

## Macrophages change with age

Among the age-related changes that occurs to macrophages is a decline in their phagocytic (identifying and dissolving) ability which has been observed in multiple tissues including the peritoneum (lining of the abdominal cavity) [122], lungs [123], bone marrow [124] and brain [125].

This dysfunction is a consequence of several different factors including senescence [126], defective autophagy [127], reduced NAD availability [128], and impairments in mitochondrial functions such as reduced ATP production, the electrical potential across the mitochondrial membrane and increased reactive oxygen species production [129,130].

Dry fasting is much like troop replenishment. Age-related alterations in macrophage phenotypes contribute to macrophage dysfunction. They have been fighting too long. M2-like macrophages become less anti-inflammatory, less phagocytic and are reduced in some tissues as these firefighters are lost because a dry fasting 'troop replacement and resupply operation' never takes place.

Aging has also been shown to cause an increased number of bone marrow-derived macrophages that are skewed towards an M1 phenotype and display impaired phagocytosis and increased cytokine production as the immune system switches to emergency mode for the same reason above, wear and attrition.

Autoimmune illnesses, like Hashimoto's thyroiditis, starts occurring when the M1 inflammatory promoting microphages damage thyroid cells as the immune system starts going haywire [131]. This results in an increased expression of pro-inflammatory genes and a result of the age-related reduction of available NAD. Without it your cells can't activate sirtuins to remove the epigenetic promoters [132]. Hashimoto's can be improved with dry fasting because during a dry fast bone marrow stem cells replace the old immune system with fresh new cells as well as the restoration of the gut wall. This is like the old human resource departments saying, 'sometimes the best way to improve productivity is to fire all the lazy people'.

**Macrophages depend on mitochondria**
Inside macrophage cells are little power plants that create ATP – the energy of life. Mitochondria are dynamic organelles attached to walker proteins that

move around inside the cell on micro tubules that form an interconnected protein network: the cytoskeleton. Mitochondria lie at the central hub for cellular metabolism in their role as ATP generators and signaling propagators either through the release of proteins, metabolites, and reaction oxygen species, or as a scaffold for signaling complexes [133]. It has also been shown that mitochondrial dysfunction causes induction of stress responses, bolstering the idea that mitochondria chemically communicate their fitness to the rest of the parts of the macrophage cell they are in.

Healthy functioning mitochondria are essential for proper metabolism. Mitochondrial dysfunction contributes to inflammation, immunosenescence and has been linked to a myriad of diseases including cardiovascular disease, cancer, metabolic diseases, and aging [134,135,136,137]. All cells need mitochondria; they can't live or function without them and can't function well if they are damaged. Damaged mitochondria can result in a compromised immune response, disturbed ROS production, and/or senescence [138,139,140]. Although partially damaged mitochondria can undergo fission to remove dysfunctional components, more severe mitochondrial damage may necessitate its removal [141]. Mitophagy, activated by cellular autophagy, is one of many autophagic processes. Mitophagy is specifically for degradation of mitochondria to remove damaged or superfluous mitochondria while at the same time activating mitochondrial biogenesis to replace the removed ones.

Mitochondria can migrate towards lysosomes to transfer power to beneficial inflammatory processes such as breaking down worn-out macrophages [142,143]. But chronic mitochondrial stress, which occurs during unabated low-level inflammation, can impair lysosomal functions [144,145]. Lysosomal impairment leads to an accumulation of lipofuscin, an almost impossible to digest cytosol glycated sugar. Lipofuscin is particularly bad because it can further dysregulate mitochondrial function by forcing mitochondria to expend energy to the lysosome overnight to digest lipofuscin to no avail because it takes longer than a night's sleep to get lipofuscin broken down. This then wears out the lysosome while leading to impaired mitophagy (getting rid of broken mitochondria and replacing them), increased ROS production, and reduced ATP generation [146]; a vicious unavoidable metabolic circle, if eating is never paused longer than a night's sleep. Calorie restriction, vitamin E, and glutathione appear to reduce or halt the production of lipofuscin but doesn't get rid of the deposits that have already accumulated. It's a very tough sugar-lipid-protein product.

My theory is that mitophagy is impaired with age because the cellular system is never taken off-line by an extended period of autophagy to fix serious cellular issues like damaged mitochondria. Autophagic dysregulation contributes to inflammation and has been associated with several age-related diseases like sarcopenia as muscle cell mitochondria become dysfunctional. [147,148,149].

**All that being said...**

The only reason the fire fighters from the fire department (macrophages) have been activated is because the metabolic fire damage is ever increasing with age due to the ever-accumulating metabolic debris from the eating metabolism. The immune system wouldn't be in emergency mode if there weren't all the metabolic fires caused by the accumulating trash. Simply living makes the cellular trash that always leads to immunosenescence and dysfunctional macrophages.

**Dry fasting changes everything**

Interestingly, dry fasting induces a response in adipose tissue and in the liver that involves macrophages that could operationally be categorized as M2 macro-phages; the ones that display a somewhat reduced inflammatory potential and are prone to promoting tissue repair and remodeling (150). Dry fasting leads to a phenotypic switch from the M1 to the M2 type of this immune cell's composition.

Dry fasting expands the previously established concept of 'metabolic fitness' to an additional area: 'immunological fitness' that is lost in the context of metabolic dysfunction. Therefore, the metabolic inflexibility, characteristic of dysfunctional tissue, is associated with the lack of 'immunological fitness.' This

# Neogenesis

can be radically changed by managing the feeding / fasting periods in a calculated way to protect the immune system.

Being metabolically younger is being in a metabolic state where the fire department is only rescuing kittens from trees.

# The Apex Omnivores Dilemma

*"Don't eat anything your great grandmother wouldn't recognize as food"*
-Michael Pollan

# 9

# Ancient Food vs Modern Food

*50,000 years ago, you needed to wake up and get ready for the days hunt. You had to have energy stored somewhere in the body from the food you ate and the muscularity to use it, because you and your fellow hunters determined whether your tribe survived. And you may have to trek far and wide...*

# Neogenesis

## The food that got us here

L Amber O'Hearn, researcher and speaker on carnivory, is also of the same opinion as Dr. Thompson that the Homo species got their start as lipovores, not carnivores. Our scavenging and breaking of bones of large animals from predatory kills to find food was to find the most energy dense means of sustenance, fat. Animal fat is your oldest and most reliable friend, it always has been. At our beginning it was both our solution to survive and, as an offshoot, it grew our brains to invent better ways to compete with the mega carnivores of that time.

We adopted meat and bone marrow to start our much earlier brain size increase, and was added to our plant-based diet, it didn't replace it. When plant food was scarce, meat gave us the ability to survive famine. Meat gave us the means to have the strength to chase and catch food as well as outrunning the predators trying to catch us as food. Meat provides us the right fatty acids that doesn't build visceral fat, in and around our liver and organs, and plant foods like tubers gave us the micronutrient minerals to operate our cellular systems better. Meat is a protein source that provides the correct ratio of amino acids and has a low omega-6 content (if it's not been corn fed). We have evolved from eating meat to have a digestive system and GI tract that is both acidic [stomach] and alkaline [intestines] to be the omnivore we are. We need macro nutrients, and micronutrients like mineral elements that are co-factors that make the co-enzymes work and most of these are found in meat as well as the other foods we eat as apex omnivore predators.

**The protein dilemma**

We as a species would have never got here to have this discussion without eating complete proteins and saturated fat. Steric and palmitic acid in meat are 16 and 18 carbon chain fatty acids. They're like a tank of high octane instead of unleaded gas when compared to plant and seed oil fatty acids. Steric and palmitic oils help your mitochondria make cellular endogenous water to flush the cell better, make more ATP and don't accumulate as visceral fat.

The problem with global health is indeed, not eating enough protein while eating unsaturated fat found in the cheapest possible industrially produced plant oils. In the western world, either by economic unavailability or psychological programming, we are eating less meat proteins than ever before. Why?

During the 1980's the PETA movement started. A global change in consciousness that was absolutely necessary for stopping the cruelty surrounding animal food production. But as always, the law of unintended consequences started a movement away from meat toward veganism that strived to replace meat by providing plant-based protein alternatives.

However, I believe in choice as much as in ethical abstinence. You can eat anything you want but I eat for life extension and metabolic function and try to avoid foods that hurt that goal.

# Neogenesis

## Modern food

Our modern diet was developed by 'experts' in nutrition. And it's been largely focused on grains, eating a 'rainbow' of different plant foods and lots of carbohydrates. Not protein and fat. The low-fat craze, the low salt craze, corn oil, margarine or the idea that 'fat makes you fat' mantra for instance, that the 'experts' promoted, has done incalculable damage to global health.

> *"We are not living longer we are dying longer."*
> -Dr. Joel Fuhrman

Another problem in the food supply is the de-mineralization of crop land by over harvesting resulting in mineral depletion. As seen in this chart; as minerals in food decrease, illness's increase.

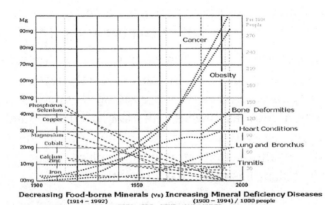

**Decreasing Food-borne Minerals (vs) Increasing Mineral Deficiency Diseases**
(1914 – 1992)        (1900 – 1994) / 1000 people
USDA – CDC – NCHS – AHA - NHNES

The practice of using industrial chemicals to grow food is killing the life in the soil and producing nutrient deficient food.

# Neogenesis

As seen in the image below you would have to eat 24 or more apples today to get the same amount of iron as in 1 apple in 1950.

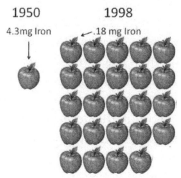

And this doesn't begin to address the contamination of our food by chemical pesticides, herbicides, and fungicides and the wide variety of toxic chemicals that are sprayed on genetically modified crops. Today the industry even sprays glyphosate on non-genetically modified crops to dry them out prior to harvest. Pre-harvest crop desiccation. Originating in Scotland in the 1980s, this practice involves applying glyphosate to a standing crop toward the end of the growing season with the express purpose of expediting the natural process where a crop slowly dies and dries in the field [166]. This is now commonly used on wheat. And a large part of our health is negatively affected by what Dr. Joe Mercola calls mitochondrial toxic fatty acids...linoleic acid found in plants. The highest levels are in borage oil is 38.47%, in evening primrose oil is 74%, in canola oil 20.12%, in corn oil 59.27%, in sunflower oil 71.17%, in cottonseed oil 56.35%, in linseed oil 15.18%, in soybean oil 56%

## The plant and seed oil dilemma

The use of industrial vegetables oils; canola, corn and soy and seed oils like safflower and cottonseed, for instance, along with high fructose corn syrup in almost all processed foods, has caused an epidemic in obesity and digestive dysfunction. Our genetic programming to seek out sources of food that create fat for reserve energy makes it almost impossible to avoid this toxic food. Almost all modern processed food has such a high glycemic index it is almost impossible not to gain excess weight nor avoid overtaxing your pancreas to keep you alive; despite your 'good' eating habits. Gluten free food replacements for wheat like tapioca flour, rice flour or beet flour have a higher glycemic index than actual cane sugar.

## Our dilemma is finding safe food

It's a bit harder to find safe food during this time of food production in human history. It may be convenient to go to a supermarket any time of day, but what you'll typically find will be genetically modified, chemically grown produce (unless you are specifically shopping at an organic grocer) and shelves full of processed foods, each with an ingredient lists of chemical additives, sweeteners, artificial flavors, and coloring. And last but certainly not least high linoleic content industrial oils; safflower, cottonseed, canola, corn, and soy.

## Navigating the mine field of industrialized meat

There are significant issues surrounding the industrialization of the meat today, not the least of which is the inhumane treatment these animals suffer their entire life. Cows are sent to a Concentrated Animal Feeding Operation (CAFO) to be fattened up for the last six months of their life by feeding them GMO corn, liquified fat, protein, alfalfa often sprayed with glyphosate before harvest, silage, and drugs. It's politely called 'marbling the meat', but fat deposits that accumulate this rapidly are the result of a desperate attempt by the animal to get the corns' 60% linoleic fatty acids out of the blood stream and into fat cells in tissue to stay alive. This is because their digestive system can't tolerate corn; it destroys their liver and rumen and makes them sick, at which time they are slaughtered for human consumption. But it does make the cow weigh more for a higher price. So yes, for the economic benefit, the meat industry condones illness in cattle. So logically this means if you are NOT eating grass fed, grass finished beef, you are likely eating the meat from a sick animal, loaded with all the wrong oils in the 'marbling'. This same flagrant cruelty applies to the chicken and hog industry. Not to mention that the enormous amount of animal waste produced by these huge operations contaminate the local aquafers and wells.

**Facts are stubborn things**

The sad fact is that modern man is losing ground. I put a chart in an earlier chapter of our brain size growth history, and indeed modern mans' brain size is decreasing.

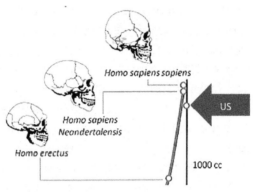

Could it be the food?

> *"You're not going to die from secondhand smoke, SARs, or monkey pox, **it's the food**. The call is coming from inside the house. The killer is not west Nile, or Avian flu, or shark attacks, it's the buffalo wings. It's the aspartame, it's the Nutra sweet, and the red dye number 2, and the high fructose corn syrup, and the MSG and the chlorine, and whatever the shit is in the 'special sauce'. It's the steroids, it's the hormones and antibiotics that are in the beef. I wouldn't touch a hot dog even if you put a condom on it. We feed cows too sick to stand to people too fat to walk. And then we wonder how these diseases spring up. Like mad cow and AIDs and Ebola. You know nature doesn't ask a lot, it really doesn't. Don't grind up the cattle and fed it to the cattle, and don't fuck the monkeys. These aren't big requests.*
>
> *-Bill Maher*

# Neogenesis

**Nutrient requirements for health**

The simplest of the competing nutrition theories seems to be that meat is what you are, so eat what you are. Well, our muscles are meat, but the facts say you also need nutrients not found in meat.

To be consistent with our genetic evolution we need to eat several sources of protein laden foods, (plant or animal), which can be found in a wide variety of foods because we need protein for its amino acids. Meat is only one of the many sources of amino acids that we've come across. Plant protein sources that contain the 9 essential amino acids, (histidine, isoleucine, leucine, lysine, methionine, phenylalanine, threonine, tryptophan, and valine) are diverse, like hemp seed hearts, amaranth, quinoa, or spirulina. We also need micronutrient mineral elements. The abundance of minerals we need come in plants, extracted from soil – our direct connection with the Earths microbiome. Eating soil grown organic food is my preferred plant food.


The bottom line is this. Neogenesis is not about what you should or shouldn't eat. It's about rethinking food, to consider what foods will do for you

…or to you.

# Neogenesis

Neogenesis

# 10

## What to do...What to do

*"Don't buy food products with more than five ingredients or any ingredients you can't easily pronounce,"*

-Michael Pollan

# Neogenesis

**Basic tenet of Neogenesis– eat everything – sort of...**
It doesn't matter if you're a meat eater, vegetarian or vegan, the only concern is eating food that doesn't mess with your endocrine system or act as anti-nutrients preventing absorption.

Your dietary protein must have enough of the amino acid leucine to activate mTOR and food that has enough saturated fatty acids for the correct lipids to drive the ATP machine without gumming up the works.

Neogenesis is a way to rethink food and daily life based on the current physiological and psychological knowledge of eating and mental health as it relates to our evolution.  But if you perform The Phoenix Protocol 7-day dry fast yearly your concerns about food should be dramatically reduced. Any damage or toxic exposure during the 51 weeks of eating will likely be repaired during the 1 week of dry fasting.

**What to do**
Right off the bat try to avoid getting most of your calories from simple sugars and choose complex carbohydrates to avoid insulin spikes. Go back to what you are; a protein/fat/tuber eater with seasonal tasty berries, fruits and nuts thrown in for variety.  Eating a sub optimal amount of protein daily has led to the epidemic of sarcopenia. The minimum amount of protein needed per day is 1.5 grams per kilograms. If you are 150 pounds (68kg), you need around 100 grams (3.5oz) of the correct source of amino acids in protein.

But you can also achieve this by taking amino acid supplements [137,138]. Anything less than this amount will lead to the slow erosion of your muscles.

*"We are not overweight; we are under muscled."*
-Dr. Gabrielle
Lyons

I explained why you need strong bones, but why do you need muscle? Because muscle is the largest organ in the body, and the one that that burns glucose; it can control your weight without dieting. Muscle mass protects all the organs, protects bones from fracture and it burns fat even at rest. And literally, 'you can't leave home without it!'

*"We have no requirement for carbohydrates.*
*We have an absolute requirement for protein."*
-Dr. Donald Layman

**Why not eat lots of carbs?**
Carbs make energy in the form of glucose. Glucose stimulates the pancreas to make insulin to drive the glucose into muscle cells to power the muscles. If you're making more glucose than your muscles can process, the excess glucose will be taken out of the blood and put into adipose tissue – to save your life. This natural process prevents a sugar coma for one thing, but this is also why it's so easy to get fat. There's no other outcome because that's how the body is designed for survival.

The other side of the coin is that overeating carbs over stimulates the pancreas to make enough insulin in response to all the glucose creating hyperinsulinemia.

105

# Neogenesis

This is where the body contains too much insulin, a condition with links to insulin resistance, diabetes and a host of other damage to body systems and organs [53,54,55,61,62,64].

The objective of Neogenesis is to build the physical body into a state of metabolic invincibility for living over vast lengths of time – a philosophy of time travel if you will.

**It's your choice**
You almost can't screw this up, but you might want to eat some safer, organic, food most of the time. It will certainly improve your odds. Support your local farmer's market by purchasing their fresh, nutrient laden organically grown food. They are a dwindling population due to big Ag and big tech investors buying up small farms.

But ultimately this changes the question of 'what to eat' to 'what do I eat to stay healthy:

> *"Do you want to set your body up as a fat builder, or do you want to set your body up to be a fat burner?"*
>
> *-Dr. Christian Assad*

Trust me you want to be a fat burner. Neogenic eating is pretty easy. It's an anti-insulinogenic regime to keep insulin under control by mostly timed eating that is coordinated with exercise. This will automatically get adipose tissue formation under control, and you really

can mostly eat whatever you want; ***everything, 'except'***
***those foods that spike insulin or damage mitochondria.***

High insulin-stimulating foods like refined sugar creates
spikes in insulin that damages organs, builds fat and
takes      a      toll      on      the      whole      body
[53,54,55,56,57,59,58,60,61,62,64].

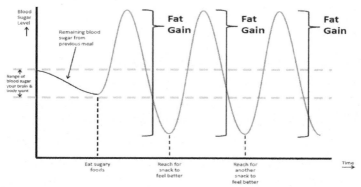

In nature the availability of high sugar content fruit,
honey and root vegetables is naturally limited. They're
ripe only over a few months, not all year. And never are
they as sugar laden as a soft drink or a candy bar. But
that's the only rule I suppose, no high insulin stimulating
food. I can assure you this gets easier as you adopt it.
Because, as you'll discover, (or already know if you've
read The Phoenix Protocol) dry fasting eliminates the
parasites that hijack your brain with chemical signals to
make you 'want' to eat all the wrong food that create
fat. Food cravings go away, and weight is subsequently
easier to control.

# Neogenesis

Sanity is more important than diet. It may take a little time to get the body you want but be patient.

*"Everywhere is within walking distance*
*if you have enough time."*

-Steven Wright

If I'm right you will have more time so, no hurries, no worries. Besides, you're here to enjoy life. I'm trying to open a path to have more of it.

## Eating like an apex omnivore predator

It's not a joke, you ARE an apex omnivore predator that has evolved to eat ANYTHING - be the omnivore. But you need to be diligent in selecting foods now-a-days.

I eat red meat, just not all the time; I also eat eggs, sardines, wild caught salmon, and free-range chickens' that peck around all day in the dirt. Again, targeted variety is the key to activating longevity genes. However, if you're a vegan or vegetarian you do need to concern yourself with consuming enough sources of essential amino acids. I mentioned spirulina and quinoa, but there are a lot of non-animal amino acid bearing foods. You don't 'need' meat you need amino acids.

Eating meat is what got us here sooner because meat has stearic acid, but all the other plant food we eat 'rounds out' our food intake for our genetics and cells to operate. Meat is just easy.

# Neogenesis

**Eating the right oils**

Stearic acid (C18:0) is a long chain dietary saturated fatty acid that has been shown to reduce metastatic tumor burden. Stearic acid is more abundant in animal fat (up to 30%) than in vegetable fat (typically <5%). The important exceptions are the foods, cocoa butter (34%) and shea butter, where the stearic acid content (as a triglyceride) is 28–45%. There is growing evidence that visceral fat is related to metastasis and decreased survival. Dietary stearic acid reduces visceral fat. In laboratory tests, lean body mass was increased in the stearic acid fed group and visceral fat was reduced by ~70% in the same group with increased monocyte chemotactic protein-1 (MCP-1); one of the key chemokines (chemical signals) that regulate migration and infiltration of macrophages into tissue to do their work [122]. Vegetable oils do exactly the opposite. So, if you choose vegetarianism or veganism, pay close attention to the oils you use for food preparation. Many plant oils stimulate macrophages to switch to M1 inflammation type macrophages, while steric acid signals M1 macrophages to switch to M2 macrophages that are anti-inflammatory and promote healing.

As I said earlier, migration of macrophages, from the blood stream across the vascular endothelium, is required for routine immunological surveillance of tissues; to root out senescent cells and toxins. Stearic acid increases this ability of these fire fighters to eliminate the sources of inflammation.

Dietary stearic acid also leads to dramatically reduced visceral fat because it stimulates apoptosis (cell death) of preadipocytes preventing the building of cells into fat tissue. Yet stearic acid, unlike the other long-chain SFAs, has no effect on blood serum levels of LDL or HDL cholesterol levels in adults.

**Apigenin**
Apigenin is a major plant flavone that has antioxidant, anti-inflammatory, and anticancer properties affecting several molecular and cellular targets as an NAD facilitator. Resveratrol also stimulates more production of NAD and that's one supplement I suggest taking daily (*see page 144*). Foods like parsley, chamomile, celery, spinach, artichokes, and oregano increase available NAD+ levels and act as anti-mutagens because of this characteristic. The microbiome-feeding fermented apigenin's like sauerkraut and pickles also provide probiotics and vitamin K2 [124]. Pharmacokinetically, they stay in the system longer which keeps their effects working.

Another apigenin is Fisetin, which I highly recommend and take daily to rid the body of senescent cells (*see page 144*).

**What not to do: high fat diets**
Fasting increases adiponectin levels, whereas lipid loading (high fat diet) leads to a reduction in adiponectin levels. Adiponectin is involved in regulating glucose levels as well as fatty acid breakdown in adipose tissue.

# Neogenesis

In fasted mice studies, lipid loading reduced adiponectin levels. Adiponectin shifts macrophages toward an M2 phenotype; the ones that are anti-inflammatory [120]. If you want more inflammation, eat more fat. Naturally I do not recommend a high fat diet.

**Your choice: modern man or a cave man?**
For instance, if you eat the modern standard American diet (SAD), you will be a fat builder and become overweight with health problems. A day or two per month of eating totally healthy foods will not change your body at all. You will still have your SAD body after eating healthy food.

Conversely, if you eat a caveman diet you will become a fat burner and get your weight under control and improve your metabolic profile. You can eat and drink and indulge in any vice for several days per month with NO significant impact on your improved metabolic profile.

It's always a good idea to feed yourself clean, high-quality food, but at the same time realize that after the first dry fast, the burden on cellular metabolism from stored toxins has been removed. You just can't re-accumulate 20, 40, 60 years of toxins and metabolic debris in a year. So, your food choices can be made with less concern.

Look, after years of research and removing all the commercial interests and hidden agendas behind most of the advice we hear, using your own metabolic capabilities strategically is the simplest way to last longer in a younger body. This is the essence of Neogenesis.

Based on my experience I'm confident that if you dry fast a week per year and severely limit the foods that age you and add a little exercise (like 3 minutes a day) this will be the path out of the scary woods of certain death at 80 years old.

### It's all about perspective

The perspective of most health 'experts' is based on two generally accepted ideas; that you must eat every day and that people will die.

But as Donald Rumsfeld once said, *"you don't know what you don't know"*. And you now know that if you dry fast, it completely changes the game. The current advice about healthy living does extend health span but never radically extends lifespan.

But their advice is still good advice, because it can be applied to Neogenesis as a force multiplier, just like applying dry fasting is a force multiplier by using its regeneration benefits when you're not sick.

### Self-control needs guidelines

That being said, for the most part there is no 'one size fits all' regarding nutrition, but there are some reasonable guidelines to keep in mind. Just about everyone can wrap their head around these ideas and if you incorporate them, you lose fat, gain muscle mass, and have an improved metabolic profile. This philosophy can be distilled into five reasonable suggestions (that I'll discuss in detail in Chapter 11) that incorporate how we had to live to 'harden up' before the 'modern world' made everything so darn convenient. Convenience is hurting us now, making us weaker mentally and physically.

**Here are the Neogenesis '5 pillars of life extension'.**

1. *Restrict carbs most of the time*
2. *Consume enough protein daily*
3. *Restrict your daily eating window*
4. *Weight resistance training*
5. *Get cold regularly*

*And don't forget...*

### **Break the rules on the weekend**
*(Celebrate life for mental health)*

Taking this to its logical conclusion, you can eat just about anything by correctly scheduling the eating and not-eating metabolisms during the year.

I think this perspective makes life easier and longer and, with a little exercise, makes you a lot more durable.

# Neogenesis

# 11

# The Neogenesis Guidelines

*"Ah, well you see the Pirate Code
is more what you'd call "guidelines" than
actual rules."*

-Capt. Hector Barbossa

# Neogenesis

## 1 - Restrict carbs most of the time

Controlling food that have carbohydrates, often in the form of sucrose, fructose, or galactose, will automatically control insulin production, protect the pancreas, and increases the ability to become a fat burner. Eating foods that stimulate the over production of insulin can only result in fat deposition, pancreatic damage, and insulin insensitivity.

## 2 - Consume enough protein daily

Many plant proteins are digestible into amino acids, but plant-based proteins are less digestible than animal proteins [50]. Plant-based proteins have less of an anabolic effect than animal proteins due to their lower digestibility, lower essential amino acid content (especially leucine), and deficiency in other essential amino acids, such as sulfur-based amino acids or lysine. Thus, plant amino acids are directed toward oxidation rather than used for muscle protein synthesis [161]. Several studies have evaluated the effect of consuming plant-based proteins on muscle protein metabolism in young, adult and old rats, pigs, and humans, compared to animal proteins, i.e., meat, milk, and its constitutive proteins (casein and whey proteins) [19,20,21,22,23,24,25,26,27,28,29,30,31,32,33,34,35,36,37,38,39,40,41,42,43,44]. A few of these studies have focused on the impact of plant-based foods [41], soy protein [42,43], or wheat protein [44] ingestion on protein synthesis at the whole body or skeletal muscle level in older individuals. Most of these studies have reported that good-quality animal proteins have a greater ability to enhance muscle protein synthesis rate and support muscle mass than plant-based proteins. But worldwide, more people eat plant-based proteins than animal-based protein [45]. Plant-based diets are not just valuable for physical human health including decreased risk of developing cancers, type 2 diabetes and cardiovascular diseases but are also more environmentally sustainable than animal-based diets, as recently reviewed by Lynch et al. [46].

Meat protein is my preferred go to food for the highest nutrient density and ratio of fat to protein. The big issue with meat is how it's grown. It must be grass fed and grass finished and never had a hoof in a feed lot eating glyphosate-soaked corn. Sardines and red meat are the best protein sources for all the amino acids followed by eggs and spirulina.

The average human body needs a minimum of 100 grams of protein per day. Dr. Gabrielle Lyons suggests 1 to 1.5 grams per kilo of body weight, and I follow her guideline; especially since my concern is maintaining and building muscle mass to prevent sarcopenia. This protein requirement can go up significantly depending on demand, body building method, endurance training or a movie role to look like Thor.

### 3 – Restrict your daily eating window
Time restricted eating in an 8-hour window of 11am to 7pm is ideal because if you stop eating by 7pm blood sugar levels will normalize before sleep.

# Neogenesis

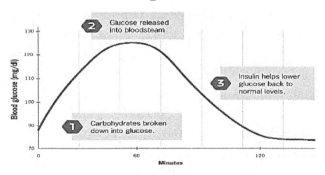

Blood level changes in insulin after eating

At night the pineal gland secretes melatonin into the bloodstream and has various effects in the body, inducing sleep, reducing our core body temperature, and inhibiting the release of insulin. Insulin is produced by the beta cells of the pancreas. These beta cells express a receptor for melatonin: the MT1 melatonin receptor. When levels of melatonin in the bloodstream are high during the night, melatonin binds to the MT1 receptor and suppresses the secretion of insulin by pancreatic beta cells. As a result, your circulating levels of insulin drop overnight if you don't pack on the food before bed. Stopping eating hours before bed causes levels of insulin and glucose circulating in your bloodstream to fall but not all the glucose. A steady overnight supply of glucose in the blood is required by your brain, which is very active during sleep and requires glucose to stay alive. The blood requires glucose for fuel and will keep transporting oxygen to the cells to keep the rest of the body alive during sleep.

# Neogenesis

Unlike other tissues, skeletal muscle, brain cells and red blood cells don't require insulin to take up glucose from the bloodstream for fuel. By inhibiting insulin secretion during sleep, melatonin helps to keep blood glucose levels adequately high, ensuring your brain is well fueled during the night because there is no insulin moving glucose into muscle and a higher blood serum level of glucose is available to the brain and blood. High glucose levels, by eating right before bed, will cause you to go to the bathroom all night, resulting in inconsistent sleep patterns. Good deep sleep is essential for longevity. How to maintain the pineal glands melatonin secretion? We talked about it earlier...get enough tryptophan in your diet.

### 4 - Weight resistance training

*"The best exercise is the one you actually do."*

Weight resistance exercise builds muscle and bone to prevent sarcopenia and osteoporosis, improves posture and helps you sleep better.

As I said earlier, exercise and strength training cause a newly identified bone derived hormone (osteocalcin) to be created. It only has minor effects on bone mineralization and density, but it's been discovered that it controls several physiological processes as a hormone that affects glucose homeostasis and exercise capacity, brain development, hippocampus integrity, cognition as well as male and female fertility.

## 5 - Get cold regularly

Brown fat has more mitochondria that white fat [167]. These mitochondria produce heat due to a unique uncoupling protein; uncoupling protein 1 (UCP1) [166]. It helps mitochondria in brown fat catalyze fatty acids to produce heat energy instead of primarily ATP. Ending every hot shower with cold water, and cycling it – 20 seconds hot, 20 seconds cold, etc., is a beneficial hormetic stress to stimulate white fat cells to transform into brown fat cells. Because your body MUST maintain a temperature of 98.6 it will go to great lengths to maintain that temperature. You can certainly keep your indoor temperature lower and sleep in a cooled room at night (65F), but these are air temperature applications, and air is not as efficient at thermal exchange as water. And there are other cold-water methods that I suggest.

- *Drink ice cold water all day*

- *Immerse your face in a sink full of ice water for 30 seconds.*
   *Paul Newman did this every morning to keep his skin taut.*

- *Cold showers daily*

- *Cold weather workouts in thin clothes with as much skin as*
   *possible exposed.*

Brown fat mitochondria will go into high heat generation and white fat will supply fatty acids to the brown fat mitochondria to keep core body temperature stable. The same for swimming in unheated pools; why do you think Olympic gold medalist Michael Phelps can eat a 12,000-calorie diet during training? Is it because he's swimming in an unheated pool all day?

All that being said...

**Break the rules at least one day per week**
I don't know about you, but I would go nuts if I couldn't enjoy a nice bottle of Merlot, some brie cheese and a baguette from time to time.

But I think you'll find that once you adopt Neogenesis and your body gets stronger and younger, there is less desire to let it all hang out and do pub crawls.

# Neogenesis

# 12

## The 'Other' You

*Thinking is a cascade of neurochemical events, and the microbiome creates many of our neurochemicals. The total microbiome weighs as much as your brain.*
*What came first? The biome or the brain?*

# Neogenesis

## The significance of insignificance

You might think that microorganisms are so small they are insignificant. Humans foolishly believe that they have conquered the earth because they think they can destroy it. Nothing could be further from the truth.

*Scientists have revealed a massive biosphere of life hidden under the Earth's Surface* [162].

> *"The deep biosphere is an abundant source of countless life-forms – totaling some 15 to 25 billion tons of microorganisms (between 245 to 385 times greater than the equivalent mass of all humans on the surface)."*

The deep biosphere of earth will always survive.

## Worship the ground you walk on

Once upon a time, under the ground you walk on, only fungi and bacteria inhabited the earth. Make no mistake, they are still here. The first kingdom conquered this planet 2.5 billion years before any plants arrived on the scene. Through conditions that would not allow any plant or animal life; bacteria and fungi...thrived. In fact, they turned our early non breathable atmosphere into the one we now enjoy. Over untold number of asteroid impacts, ice ages, magnetic field reversals, volcanic eruptions, toxic atmospheric and oceanic conditions, solar flares, coronal mass ejections, solar micro nova bursts and the cosmic radiation that mutated them, the first order of life above and below the surface...survived.

# Neogenesis

Over time, it is thought that evolution resulted in the higher kingdoms of life. But the survival of the 'higher' forms of life are completely dependent on the first kingdom organisms. Their microscopic biological metabolic synthesis of nutrients into biologically active compounds makes the micro biome essential in soil for plants as well as in the gut for the animal kingdom.

## It's better to be first

The first kingdom is necessary for more complex life to exist on this planet; it's the microorganisms that provide for the life to exist in these 'higher' orders. We could not live without them. Our mothers pass their microbiome to their infants at birth via the birth canal. It's now a common practice to swab cesarean born babies with the mother's vaginal fluids to assure healthy neonatal development.

But once the higher order organisms die...they are consumed by, and there after returned to, the first order.

Which begs the question: is this idea that we are the most complex and evolved life form on earth...an illusion?  Is our perceptual reality, 'thought', manufactured by the 'hive mind' generated by the population inside the biological condominium that you physically are?  Our human biome has 100 times more organisms than the number of cells in our physical body; 100 trillion body cells compared to 10,000 trillion microorganisms. Which came first, the chicken or the egg? Biome or the being?

A perplexing idea, eh?

Parasites can affect your food selections; bacteria can deplete amino acids and minerals that affect your mood and psyche...happiness and focus are based on a happy, in-balance gut micro biome.

A strong, balanced gut micro biome population is essential for what I am calling functional immortality. There is unity in strength and strength in unity.

**Who are we...really?**
Simply put, we evolved from plants that in turn evolved with organisms in soil. Was it the earths biome that invented the higher orders? Plant's live well (or not) based on the quality of the life in the soil, the soil microorganisms. You derive nutrients manufactured from the microorganisms inside your gut, which is in every way your soil, and you live well or not because of the quality of the life living in your soil - your gut. Feeding your biome correctly will directly affect your quality of life.

> *"The road to good health is paved with good intestines."*
>
> *-Dr. Sherry Rogers*

The first thing to realize is that you are a carbon/calcium-based bio photon activated, genetic code operating system, chemical factory that provides a condominium for your micro biome. That condominium is either well maintained or rotting from the inside out and damaged daily...by habit or user error.

You are not just 'you'. You are the vast number of living beings that allow 'you' to live and rely on you to provide a movable dwelling so both of you can live. It's a partnership. And they have been here for 3.5 billion years when the red algae in the primordial oceans were transformed by cosmic radiation into oxygen-producing green algae; this alone took a billion years. You, the plants, and other animals are just an apartment complex for the first order of life.

They were here first, and they conquered this planet billions of years ago. I sometimes wonder if they 'invented' us just to carry them around...over the land, in the air, into space, to the moon and soon to Mars.

**The gut brain connection**
We have a specialized organ, the mesentery. Anatomically, it's a fold of skin inside the peritoneum which enwraps and attaches the stomach, small intestine, pancreas, spleen, and other organs to the posterior wall of the abdomen. Neurologically, it's a huge and complex bio-wiring harness of nerves, blood, PVS, and lymphatic vessels that wraps around the intestines. It monitors and coordinates the chemical and electrical information sent between the gut and the brain by chemicals produced by the biome in the interior gut wall.

# Neogenesis

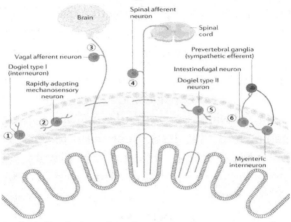

These chemical signals stimulate the system of nerves that monitor the chemicals produced in the cells of the gut epithelium for the brain via the vagus nerve. It's a very specifically designed fascial matrix architecture 'wiring harness' permeating the gut, facilitating information shared with the brain. It, arguably, may make it the most important organ in the body. It's like the radar tower operating the air traffic control system making sure jets don't crash into each other or miss the airport altogether.

A couple of words you have likely never heard of are 'plexus' and 'lumen.' A lumen is the inside space of a tubular structure, such as the interior wall of an artery or the intestine. It comes from the Latin 'an opening.' A plexus is a complex of nerves and vessels in the body.

This is clearly seen in the integration of the nervous system inside the mesentery submucosal plexus that provides the conduit for the blood, lymph, PVS and nerves that wraps around the intestines. This organ is the means of sensing changes in the intestinal lumen to monitor and keep the nutrient extraction and processing system of the digestive system operating flawlessly.

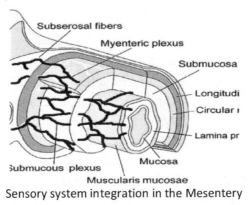

Sensory system integration in the Mesentery

Mucosae are the linings of the tubes and are in layers, The submucous plexus lies in the submucosa of the intestinal wall. The nerves of this plexus are the black lines penetrating all layers in the image above. One layer reporting information to the next layer inside of outer layers. The myenteric plexus holds the major nerve supply to the gastrointestinal tract. It provides nerve signals to the submucosa glands that produce lubricants (mucus) to move materials through the intestines. This very complex layered system contains fascial sensors that monitor everything going on in the lumen, connected with chemical signals inside the mucosa to report back to the brain

Hunger can activate these nerves to stimulate chemical interventions during fasting and ketosis.

# Neogenesis

**It's a closed loop system.**
The lumen microorganisms are monitored by the blood and brain and the brain is monitored by the chemicals in the blood produced by organisms in the lumen. There is no YOU, there is only US. Without the microbiome there would be no YOU.

**How food is grown matters most in the gut**
Moreover, the immune system controls the composition of the gut microbiota, and at the same time, resident microbes provide signals that foster normal immune system development and regulate ensuing immune responses. Therefore, it is critical to not expose the intestinal microbiota to Ag chemicals like glyphosate which is specifically designed to corrupt the shikimate pathway; a seven-step metabolic pathway used by bacteria, archaea, fungi, algae, some protozoans, and plants for the biosynthesis of folates and aromatic amino acids. Glyphosate hurts soil microbes and will do the same to the microbes in your soil - your gut environment. The shikimic acid pathway is the name of the steps in the metabolism of carbohydrates and synthesis of aromatic amino acids that ultimately give rise to the synthesis of aromatic amino acids like tryptophan, tyrosine and phenylalanine in plants.

Humans can synthesize phenylalanine into tyrosine but must obtain tryptophan from food, like bananas or egg whites; the highest source.

Glyphosate changes everything because it forces the gut bacteria to stop making aromatic amino acids and instead produce toxic phenols that capture sulfur and transport it to the liver that needs sulfur, but the phenols are released when they get there causing liver damage.

**The phantom in the hedgerow**
It's also suspected by Dr Stephanie Seneff that glyphosate can replace glycine in the glutathione molecule preventing the liver from performing detoxification via the cytochrome P-450 system (Samsel, Seneff; Surg Neurol Int. 2015; 6: 45).

Disruption of these dynamic nutrient interactions by glyphosate have far-reaching effects on host health (Hamard et al., 2007).

It is completely understood now that gut health is essential for brain health. This whole system can be interrupted by damage to the liver's cytochrome P-450 detoxification system. Interrupting this system makes it harder for the body to fight the natural and unnatural environmental chemicals that must be dealt with on a daily basis.

The health of the human biome is a major key to longevity, health and ultimately functional immortality.

# Neogenesis

# 13

## The 'Other' Other You

*The Universe is a thinking stuff from which all things are made and which, in its original state, permeates, penetrates and fills the inter spaces of the universe.*

---

*Man is a thinking mind in a thinking stuff. A thought in that substance produces the thing that is imaged by the thought.*

---

*Man can form things in his thoughts and, by his impressing them on formless substance, can cause the things he thinks about to be created."*

*-Wallace Wattles -*

*1910*

# Neogenesis

## A memory experiment

Try to remember what you think about and watch your thoughts come into existence to see this work for yourself. It's sometimes explained away as coincidence, but isn't coincidence something 'co'... 'in siding'?

Remarkably, in all of history, you are the only example of a 'thinking' thinking stuff. Proof? We've gone to the moon and back...by thinking it first...get it now? Thinking matters. 'Ya gotta be there before you get there' is one of any number of sayings to capture this fact about our universe. This has been hidden away for centuries and only used by mankind's rulers to make empires. It was written on the emerald tablets of Hermes Trismegistus.

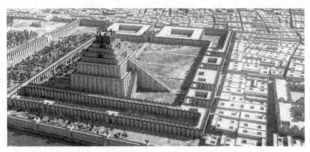

And it was written in stone 7000 years ago in Samaria

> Na - mu um mu - al li da at - na ta a
> Na ta a – tu ir te hi su – sa lil
> **Bu uk ki - pa ti- ka la mu**

Translation:

> The heart gave birth to the mind
> The mind has the power to bring things into being
> **Thought forms everything**

# Neogenesis

But recently some have re-discovered this:

### Jesus Christ
"So, I say to you; ask and you shall receive."

### The lost gospel of Thomas
"When the two become one, thought and emotion, all things become possible."

### Napoleon Hill
"Think and grow rich."

### Wallace Wattles
"Riches are achieved by thinking in a certain way."

### Henry Ford
"Whether you think you can or think you can't, you're right."

### Earl Nightingale
"We become what we think about."

### Ester Hicks (Abraham)
"Think about want you want and think about why you want it, to manifest your dreams into existence."

### Kurt Vonnegut Jr.
"We are what we pretend to be, so we must be careful about what we pretend to be"

## The Placebo Effect – the power of thought
Thought can have a powerful influence on the body, and in some cases, can even help the body heal. The mind can even sometimes trick you into believing that a fake treatment has real therapeutic results, a phenomenon that is known as the placebo effect.

# Neogenesis

The placebo effect is defined as a phenomenon in which some people experience a benefit after the administration of an inactive 'look-alike' substance or treatment. This substance, or placebo, has no known medical effect. Sometimes the placebo is in the form of a pill (sugar pill), but it can also be an injection (saline solution) or drink.

But the placebo effect is much more than just positive thinking. When this response occurs, many people have no idea they are responding to what is essentially a 'sugar pill'.

This is the power of thought in action.

A fascinating landmark placebo study found that people with osteoarthritis improved equally well regardless of whether they received a genuine surgical procedure or a sham. It is a particularly striking example of the placebo effect and implies that thought can directly influence seemingly mechanical problems [150].

## The Counterclockwise Study

In 1979, Professor Ellen Langer of Harvard University was investigating the extent to which aging is a product of our state of mind. To find out, she devised a study called 'the counter-clockwise study'. [164]

It involved taking a group of men, all age 75, that were put into a closed retreat; a duplication of the world of 1959. The question she wanted to answer was, 'if we took them back 20 years in their mind, would their bodies reflect this change?'

# Neogenesis

They agreed to live in a time capsule house for a week. They dressed in 1959 clothes, slept in replicas of their very own 1959 bedrooms, watched television from that era, and spoke about the events of 1959 in the present tense. They were put through a battery of physical and psychological tests to establish their physical and mental condition before the experiment began: hearing, vision, grip, finger length, muscle mass, bone density, physical strength, blood, hormones, flexibility, and balance.

A core element of Ellen's original experiment was the idea that our prior beliefs play a huge part in how we perceive the world, and how we perceive ourselves. By immersing the volunteers in a 1959 world, they were hoping to make them think of themselves as younger, fitter, and healthier.

At the end of the week the group was put through the same battery of physical and psychological tests.

Memory, mood, flexibility, stamina and even eyesight had improved in almost all of them. All participants tested 7 to 10 years younger in just one week.

In 2010, the BBC did a follow up study where they made another closed retreat that was designed to be 35 years earlier representing the year 1975. The music, television, magazines, and furniture were all from that year. The participants were men and women aged 78 to 88. After one week they had all reduced their age markers by 12 years. The amazing thing here was that when the participants arrived some were using walking canes and one was in a wheelchair but at the end of the week, they all walked out of the test without assistance. [165]

When asked how this was possible, they all said "they *'thought'* they were younger."

It makes a compelling case for the argument that just opening our minds to what's possible can lead to better health, whatever our chronological age.

But how do we apply this to Neogenesis? I reiterate:

> *"Whether you think you can or think you can't,*
> *you're right"*
>
> *-Henry Ford*

What happens when you start 'thinking' you can live an extended lifespan?

Since our thoughts create the abstract concept of 'time', can the simple act of 'thinking' give us more time?

It just might be the first step to achieving more time.

# Neogenesis

# Neogenesis

## *Epilogue – Endless Possibilities*

*Ever-presence will have its own set of problems, like explaining your age on your driver's license in 125 years, assuming cars exist in 2146. It may require some creative thinking to come up with solutions to this and other puzzles, but I suspect with extended lifespan comes enhanced cognition to sort this out. But remaining here in the now presents an opportunity for those prepared to embrace an extended lifespan.*

*You cannot be timid.*

*It is very likely that extending lifespan at this moment in time will present some unusually difficult situations to deal with not seen for thousands of years; not the least of which is surviving a predicted 12,000-year recurring solar micro nova that is set to pop again around 2046, some 25 years from now [152]. But now, near the end of 2021, other more pressing social issues have captured our attention; like protecting our freedom and individual rights from tyrannical governments. The jury is out on how that will resolve but have courage:*

> *"Courage is being scared as hell and saddling up anyway."*
> *-John Wayne*

*You're an apex omnivore predator, and if I'm right, you'll probably live past it.*

*But I guarantee you, in ten years you'll no more care about the news happening today than you do the senators running the Credit Mobilier Scandal around the time of the election of*

# Neogenesis

*Ulysses S. Grant, or the house of representatives running the Whiskey Ring Scandal during it.*

*The path backward just won't matter, only the path forward.*

*You must steel yourself against the stress of current events to enjoy a longer life because stress reduces lifespan. But now your life might be one without aging and in that you can take some measure of solace – a quantum of solace if you will.*

*There will be victories and setbacks but with determination, tenacity, and a bit of luck you will survive what's coming.*

*A new world order is about to be brought forth once again by the SUN. It's not quite the new world order imagined by the globalist crowd, but a new one, nonetheless.*

*All is on track for my third book, but it is 2021, and anything can happen.*

*But thankfully, I have hope...*

*August*

# Neogenesis

*"I gave men hope,*
*and so turned away their eyes from death."*

**-Prometheus**

# Neogenesis

Contact August at: PhoenixProtocol@yahoo.com

# Neogenesis

## Supplements

Neogenesis utilizes specific nutraceuticals for cellular tissue maintenance and body building.

**The cellular maintenance supplements** listed below are available at **www.cytolyfe.com**, Amazon and eBay

**1 - Fisetin 500mg -** To remove senescent cells and their toxic
cytokines to prevent collateral damage in the tissue surrounding them.
https://www.ncbi.nlm.nih.gov/pmc/articles/PMC3689181/
https://pubmed.ncbi.nlm.nih.gov/27671819/

**2 - Resveratrol 1000 -** Trans-resveratrol acts to initiate NAD synthesis.
https://www.ncbi.nlm.nih.gov/pmc/articles/PMC4875984/
https://www.mdpi.com/journal/nutrients/special_issues/Benefits_of_Resveratrol_Supplementation

**3 - Stem Cell-Regen -** Supports immune system stem cell production.
https://pubmed.ncbi.nlm.nih.gov/16522169/
https://citeseerx.ist.psu.edu/viewdoc/download?doi=10.1.1.627.1160&rep=rep1&type=pdf

**4 - Polyphenol Plus -** Mitochondria protection for optimally functioning macrophage mitochondria and neural cells by controlling reaction oxygen species production
https://www.ncbi.nlm.nih.gov/pmc/articles/PMC8025073/
https://www.ncbi.nlm.nih.gov/pmc/articles/PMC6321535/
https://www.ncbi.nlm.nih.gov/pmc/articles/PMC4875984/
https://www.ncbi.nlm.nih.gov/pmc/articles/PMC6273006/#B83-molecules-21-01243

# Neogenesis

**The body building supplements**

**1 - Inner Power** by **Life Enhancement**
A pre-workout arginine supplement to enhance blood flow to muscles at the time of work out.
*I take the Inner Power™ w/xylitol – Cherry Citrus Flavored*
Available at **www. life-enhancement.com** or Amazon


**2 - Perfect Amino** by **BodyHealth**
An amino acid complex for delivering amino acid nutrients for mTOR activation requirements to build muscle and bone.
Available at **www. bodyhealth.com** or Amazon

# Neogenesis

## References

**1 Evolution and molecular mechanisms of adaptive developmental plasticity.**
*Mol Ecol* 2011/20 1347-63

**2 Nothing in biology makes sense except in the light of evolution;**
*Am Biol Teach* 1973; 35;125–9.

**3 Phenotypic plasticity and experimental evolution.**
*J Exp Biol* 2006; 209:2344–61.

**4 Origins of the Human Predatory Pattern: The Transition to Large-Animal Exploitation by Early Hominins;**
Current Anthropology Volume 60, Number 1 February 2019

**5 Early humans used chopping tools to break animal bones and consume the bone marrow;**
Phy Org January 21, 2021

**6 Cooking and grinding reduces the cost of meat digestion.**
Comp Biochem Physiol A. Mol Integr Physiol. 2007 Nov; 148(3):651.

**7 Adriana Heguy,**
Professor of Pathology at NYU Langone Medical CenterE,

**8 Duke University Medical Center;**
medical.net/news/2007/10/08

**9 Evolution of The Human Appendix: A Biological 'Remnant' No More;**
Science daily: August 21, 2009

**10 The Mechanisms of Psychedelic Visionary Experiences: Hypotheses from Evolutionary Psychology;**
Front Neurosci. 2017; 11: 539.

**11 Revealing the paradox of drug reward in human evolution;**
https://doi.org/10.1098/rspb.2007.1673

**12 Genes and longevity: Lessons from studies of centenarians.**
J. GErontol. Ser. A Boil. Sci. Med. Sci. 2000; 55 B319-B328

**13 Genetic variation in human telomerase is associated with telomere length in Ashkenazi centenarians.**
Proc. Natl. Acad. Sci. USA/ 2010; 107: 1710-1717

**14 Disease variants in genomes of 44 centenarians.**
Mol. Genet. Genom. Med. 2014; 2: 438-450

# Neogenesis

15 Impact of telomerase ablation on organismal viability, aging, and tumorigenesis in mice lacking the DNA repair proteins PARP-1, Ku86, or DNA-PKcs.
J. Cell Boil. 2004; 167:627–638.

16 Shorter telomeres are associated with mortality in those with APOE ε4 and dementia.
Ann. Neurol. 2006; 60:181–187.

17 The Rate of Increase of Short Telomeres Predicts Longevity in Mammals. Cell Rep. 2012; 2: 732-737

18 Questioning causal involvement of telomeres in aging.
Aging Res. Rev. 2015; 24: 191-196

20 Association of longer telomeres with better health in centenarians. Journals
Geronol. Ser. A: Boil. Sci. Med. Sci. 2008; 63: 809-812

21 Possible Mechanisms for Telomere Length Maintenance in Extremely Old People.
Hered, Genet. 2014; 3: 1-2

22 Decreased epigenetic age of PBMCs from Italian semi-supercentenarians and their offspring.
Aging. 2015; 7: 1159-1170

23 Evolution in health and medicine Sackler colloquium: Genetic variation in human telomerase is associated with telomere length in Ashkenazi centenarians.
Proc. Natl. Acad. Sci. USA. 2010; 107:1710–1717.

24 Association of longer telomeres with better health in centenarians
Journals Gerontol. Ser. A: Boil. Sci. Med Sci. 2008; 63:809–812.

25 Mechanisms for Telomere Length Maintenance in Extremely Old People
Hered. Genet. 2014; 3:1–2

26 Decreased epigenetic age of PBMCs from Italian semi-supercentenarians and their offspring
Aging. 2015; 7:1159–1170.

27 polymerase-1-dependent cardiac myocyte cell death during heart failure is mediated by NAD+ depletion and reduced Sirt2 deacetylase activity.
J Biol Chem 2005; 280:43121–43130

28 Exceptionally Long-Lived Individuals (ELLI) Demonstrate Slower Aging Rate Calculated by DNA Methylation Clocks as Possible Modulators for Healthy Longevity
Int J Mol Sci. 2020 Jan; 21(2): 615.

29 Fasting promotes the expression of SIRT1, an NAD$^+$-dependent protein deacetylase, via activation of PPARα in mice
*Molecular and Cellular Biochemistry* volume 339, pages285–292, 2/11/2010

30 Properties of biophotons and their theoretical implications
Indian J Exp Biol 2003 May;41(5):391-402.

31 Proteins involved in biophoton emission and flooding-stress responses in soybean under light and dark conditions
Mol Biol Rep. 2016 Feb;43(2):73-89.

32 Emission of Mitochondrial Biophotons and their Effect on Electrical Activity of Membrane via Microtubules;
https://arxiv.org/ftp/arxiv/papers/1012/1012.3371.pdf

33 Estimation of the number of biophotons involved in the visual perception of a single object image: Biophoton intensity can be considerably higher inside cells than outside;
https://arxiv.org/ftp/arxiv/papers/1012/1012.3625.pdf

34 Mitogenetic Radiation, Biophotons and Non-Linear Oxidative
Processes in Aqueous Media
Integrative Biophysics (pp.331-359)

35 Fascia: a morphological description and classification system based on a literature review
J Can Chiropr Assoc. 2012 Sep; 56(3): 179–191.

36 Bone Tissue is an Integral Part of the Fascial System;
Cureus. 2019 Jan; 11(1): e3824.

37 https://www.anatomytrains.com/fascia/

38 Extracellular Matrix (ECM)
https://fasciaguide.com/fascia-anatomy-physiology/extracellular-matrix/

39 New Proposal to Define the Fascial System
https://www.karger.com/article/fulltext/486238

40 Hyaluronan and the Fascial Frontier
*Int. J. Mol. Sci.* 2021, *22*(13), 6845

# Neogenesis

**41 TERMINOLOGY USED IN FASCIA RESEARCH**
HTTPS://FASCIACONGRESS.ORG/CONGRESS/FASCIA-GLOSSARY-OF-TERMS/

**42 Tensegrity**
https://www.anatomytrains.com/fascia/tensegrity/

**43 Anatomy, Fascia.**
https://www.ncbi.nlm.nih.gov/books/NBK493232/

**44 Fascia and Primo Vascular System**
Evidence-based Complementary and Alternative Medicine August 2015(1):1-6

**45 The Primo Vascular System as a New Anatomical System**
Journal of Acupuncture and Meridian Studies Volume 6, Issue 6, December 2013, Pages 331-338

**46 New Developments in Primo Vascular System: Imaging and Functions with regard to Acupuncture**
https://doi.org/10.1155/2015/303769

**47 mTOR and the health benefits of exercise**
Seminars in Cell & Developmental Biology, Volume 36, December 2014, Pages 130-139

**48 Geroscience: Linking aging to chronic disease**
Cell. 2014;159(4):709–13.

**49 Immunosenescence and inflamm-aging as two sides of the same coin: Friends or foes?**
Front Immunol. 2018; 8:1960

**50 The hallmarks of aging.**
Cell. 2013;153(6):1194–217.

**51 7 pillars of life extension**
https://www.24life.com/dave-asprey-why-we-need-to-be-super-human/

**52 5 tactics for longevity**
https://peterattiamd.com/the-5-tactics-in-the-longevity-toolkit/

**53 Insulin Plays Central Role in Aging**
https://www.sciencedaily.com/releases/2004/06/040603064935.htm

**54 Insulin, Aging, and the Brain: Mechanisms and Implications;**
Front Endocrinol (Lausanne). 2015; 6: 13.

**55 Age, Obesity, and Sex Effects on Insulin Sensitivity and Skeletal Muscle Mitochondrial Function**
Diabetes. 2010 Jan; 59(1): 89–97.

56 Mechanism of increased risk of insulin resistance in aging skeletal muscle
*Diabetology & Metabolic Syndrome* **volume 12**, Article number: 14 (2020)

57 Insulin Resistance Causes and Symptoms
https://www.endocrineweb.com/conditions/type-2-diabetes/insulin-resistance-causes-symptoms

58 Age-Related Changes in Glucose Metabolism, Hyperglycemia, and Cardiovascular Risk
https://doi.org/10.1161/CIRCRESAHA.118.312806

59 An eye on insulin
J Clin Invest. 2003 Jun 15; 111(12): 1817–1819.

60 Hyperglycemia induced testicular damage in type 2 diabetes mellitus rats exhibiting microcirculation impairments associated with vascular endothelial growth factor decreased via PI3K/Akt pathway
Oncotarget. 2018 Jan 12; 9(4): 5321–5336.

61 The Link Between PCOS and Diabetes
https://www.endocrineweb.com/polycystic-ovary-syndrome-pcos/link-between-pcos-diabetes

62 Sweet Treats That Can Make Tinnitus Terrible
https://www.arlingtonhearingcenterva.com/hearing-loss-articles/sweet-treats-can-make-tinnitus-terrible/

63 Bone Regulates Glucose Metabolism as an Endocrine Organ through Osteocalcin
Int J Endocrinol 2015; 2015:967673.

64 Insulin Signaling in Bone Marrow Adipocytes
*Current Osteoporosis Reports* **volume 17**, pages446–454 (2019)

65 New Insights into the Biology of Osteocalcin
Bone. 2016 Jan; 82: 42–49

66 Osteocalcin is necessary and sufficient to maintain muscle mass in older mice
Mol Metab,2016 Jul 16;5(10):1042-1047.

67 A difference of bone fracture rate and frequency to have determined in diagnosis standards
Osteoporosis, 2010, 8: 266–270

68 Proper Calcium Use: Vitamin K$_2$ as a Promoter of Bone and Cardiovascular Health;
Integr Med (Encinitas). 2015 Feb; 14(1): 34–39.

69 Osteocalcin promotes β-cell proliferation during development and adulthood through Gprc6a
Diabetes, 2014 Mar;63(3):1021-31

70 GPRC6A mediates responses to osteocalcin in β-cells in vitro and pancreas in vivo
J Bone Miner Res 2011 Jul;26(7):1680-3

71 Signaling pathway for adiponectin expression in adipocytes by osteocalcin;
Cell Signal 2015 Mar;27(3):532-44.

72 Carboxylated and uncarboxylated forms of osteocalcin directly modulate the glucose transport system and inflammation in adipocytes
Horm Metab Res 2014 May;46(5):341-7.

73 The uncarboxylated form of osteocalcin is associated with improved glucose tolerance and enhanced β-cell function in middle-aged male subjects
Diabetes Metabolism Res and Rev, 29 October 2009

74 Association of serum total osteocalcin with type 2 diabetes and intermediate metabolic phenotypes: systematic review and meta-analysis of observational evidence
Eur J Epidemiol 2015 Aug;30(8):599-614.

75 Regulation of male fertility by the bone-derived hormone osteocalcin
Mol Cell Endocrinol 2014 Jan 25;382(1):521-526.

76 Osteocalcin regulates murine and human fertility through a pancreas-bone-testis axis
J Clin Invest 2013 Jun;123(6):2421-33.

77 Osteocalcin-dependent regulation of glucose metabolism and fertility: Skeletal implications for the development of insulin resistance
J Cell Physiol 2018 May;233(5):3769-3783.

78 Positive Correlation between Serum Osteocalcin and Testosterone in Male Hyperthyroidism Patients with High Bone Turnover
Exp Clin Endocrinol Diabetes 2016 Jul;124(7):452-6.

79 Undercarboxylated osteocalcin, muscle strength and indices of bone health in older women
Bone 2014 Jul; 64:8-12.

# Neogenesis

80 Osteocalcin Signaling in Myofibers Is Necessary and Sufficient for Optimum Adaptation to Exercise
Cell Metab 2016 Jun 14;23(6):1078-1092.

81 Osteocalcin Induces Proliferation via Positive Activation of the PI3K/Akt, P38 MAPK Pathways and Promotes Differentiation Through Activation of the GPRC6A-ERK1/2 Pathway in C2C12 Myoblast Cells
Cell Physiol Biochem 2017;43(3):1100-1112.

82 Hindlimb Immobilization, But Not Castration, Induces Reduction of Undercarboxylated Osteocalcin Associated With Muscle Atrophy in Rats
J Bone Miner Res 2016 Nov;31(11):1967-1978.

83 Lower serum osteocalcin concentrations are associated with brain microstructural changes and worse cognitive performance
Clin Endocrinol (Oxf) 2016 May;84(5):756-63.

84 Association between osteocalcin and cognitive performance in healthy older adults
Age Ageing. 2016 Nov; 45(6): 844–849

85 Low serum osteocalcin concentration is associated with incident type 2 diabetes mellitus in Japanese women
J Bone Miner Metab 2018 Jul;36(4):470-477.

86 Independent Relationship of Osteocalcin Circulating Levels with Obesity, Type 2 Diabetes, Hypertension, and HDL Cholesterol\
Endocr Metab Immune Disord Drug Targets 2016;16(4):270-275.

87 Association between Serum Total Osteocalcin Level and Type 2 Diabetes Mellitus: A Systematic Review and Meta-Analysis;
Horm Metab Res 2015 Oct;47(11):813-9.

88 Low osteocalcin level is a risk factor for impaired glucose metabolism in a Chinese male population
J Diabetes Investig 2016 Jul;7(4):522-8.

89 Decreased undercarboxylated osteocalcin in children with type 2 diabetes mellitus
J Pediatr Endocrinol Metab 2016 Aug 1;29(8):879-84

# Neogenesis

102 Serum Osteocalcin Levels in Children With Nonalcoholic Fatty Liver Disease;
J Pediatr Gastroenterol Nutr 2018 Jan;66(1):117-121.

103 Inverse relationship between serum osteocalcin levels and nonalcoholic fatty liver disease in postmenopausal Chinese women with normal blood glucose levels
Acta Pharmacol Sin 2015 Dec;36(12):1497-502.

104 Association between serum osteocalcin levels and non-alcoholic fatty liver disease in women
Digestion. 2015;91(2):150-7.

105 Association of nonalcoholic fatty liver disease with bone mineral density and serum osteocalcin levels in Korean men
Eur J Gastroenterol Hepatol 2016 Mar;28(3):338-44.

106 Serum osteocalcin levels are inversely associated with the presence of nonalcoholic fatty liver disease in patients with coronary artery disease
Int J Clin Exp Med 2015 Nov 15;8(11):21435-41

107 Osteocalcin improves nonalcoholic fatty liver disease in mice through activation of Nrf2 and inhibition of JNK
Endocrine 2016 Sep;53(3):701-9.

108 Body acceleration distribution and O2 uptake in humans during running and jumping
J Appl Physiol Respir Environ Exerc Physiol 1980 Nov;49(5):881-7.

107 Central and peripheral actions of somatostatin on the growth hormone-IGF-I axis
J Clin Invest 2004 Aug;114(3):349-56.

108 Sox2(+) stem/progenitor cells in the adult mouse pituitary support organ homeostasis and have tumor-inducing potential
Cell Stem Cell 2013 Oct 3;13(4):433-45

109 Stem cell therapy and its potential role in pituitary disorders
Curr Opin Endocrinol Diabetes Obes 2017 Aug;24(4):292-300.

112 Pituitary stem cell regulation: who is pulling the strings?
J Endocrinol 2017 Sep;234(3): R135-R158.

# Neogenesis

113 **Mobilized Adult Pituitary Stem Cells Contribute to Endocrine Regeneration in Response to Physiological Demand**
Cell Stem Cell Vol 13 Issue 4 P419-432 October 03, 2013

114 **Pituitary Remodeling Throughout Life: Are Resident Stem Cells Involved?**
Front Endocrinol (Lausanne) 2021 Jan 29; 11:604519.

115 **Stress and stem cells**
Rev Dev Biol. 2012 Nov-Dec; 1(6): 10.1002/wdev.56.

116 **Inflammaging and "garb-aging"**
Trends Endocrinol Metab. 2017;28(3):199–212.

117 **Age and age-related diseases: Role of inflammation triggers and cytokines**
Front Immunol. 2018; 9:1–28.

118 **An update on inflamm-aging: Mechanisms, prevention, and treatment.**
J Immunol Res. 2016; 2016:8426874

119 **Understanding the mysterious M2 macrophage through activation markers and effector mechanisms mediators**
Inflamm 2015; 2015:1–16.

120 **Skewed macrophage polarization in aging skeletal muscle.**
Aging Cell. 2019; 18:313032

121 **Tissue-resident macrophage enhancer landscapes are shaped by the local microenvironment.**
Cell. 2014;159(6):1312–26.

122 **Aging impairs peritoneal but not bone marrow-derived macrophage phagocytosis.**
Aging Cell. 2014;13(4):699–708.

123 **Aging impairs alveolar macrophage phagocytosis and increases influenza-induced mortality in mice.**
J Immunol. 2017;199(3):1060–8.

124 **Retinoid X receptor activation reverses age-related deficiencies in myelin debris phagocytosis and remyelination**
Brain. 2015;138(12):3581–97.

125 **Microglial dysfunction in brain aging and Alzheimer's disease.**
Biochem Pharmacol. 2014;88(4):594–604.

126 Old age increases microglial senescence, exacerbates secondary neuroinflammation, and worsens neurological outcomes after acute traumatic brain injury in mice.
Neurobiol Aging. 2019; 77:194–206.

127 Autophagy controls acquisition of aging features in macrophages
J Innate Immun. 2015;7(4):375–91.

128 Macrophage de novo $NAD^+$ synthesis specifies immune in aging and inflammation.
Nat Immunol. 2019;20(1):50–63.

129 Loss of phagocytic and antigen cross-presenting capacity in aging dendritic cells Is associated with mitochondrial dysfunction
J Immunol. 2015;195(6):2624–32.

130 Clearance of apoptotic cells critically depends on the phagocyte Ucp2 protein.
Nature. 2011;477(7363):220–4.

131 Impaired phagocytosis of apoptotic cells causes accumulation of bone marrow-derived macrophages in aged mice.
BMB Rep. 2017;50(1):43–8.

132 Immunometabolism orchestrates training of innate immunity in atherosclerosis.
Cardiovasc Res. 2019;115(9):1416–24.

133 Mitochondria as signaling organelles.
BMC Biol 2014;12(1):34

134 Mitochondrial dysfunction in atherosclerosis.
Circ Res. 2007;100(4):460–73.

135 The role of mitochondria in aging
J Clin Invest. 2013;123(3):951–7.

136 Mitochondrial fission-induced mtDNA stress promotes tumor-associated macrophage infiltration and HCC progression.
Oncogene. 2019;38(25):5007–20.

137 Metabolic influences on macrophage polarization and pathogenesis.
BMB Rep. 2019;52(6):360–72.

138 Mitochondrial dysfunction contributes to oncogene-induced senescence
Mol Cell Biol. 2009;29(16):4495–507.

139 Feedback between p21 and reactive oxygen production is necessary for cell senescence
Mol Syst Biol. 2010;6(1):347

140 Mitochondrial dysfunction induces senescence with a distinct secretory phenotype.
Cell Metab. 2016;23(2):303–14.

141 Mitochondrial fission, fusion, and stress.
Science. 2012;337(6098):1062–5.

142 Function of Mitochondria–Lysosome Membrane Contact Sites in Cellular Homeostasis
Trends Cell Biol. 2019;29(6):500–13.

143 Mitochondria and lysosomes: Discovering bonds.
Front Cell Dev Biol. 2017; 5:106

144 Mitochondrial respiratory chain deficiency inhibits lysosomal hydrolysis.
Autophagy. 2019;15(9):1572–91.

145 Acute and chronic mitochondrial respiratory chain deficiency differentially regulate lysosomal biogenesis.
Sci Rep 2017;7(1):45076

146 Mitochondrial turnover and aging of long-lived postmitotic cells: The mitochondrial–lysosomal axis theory of aging.
Antioxid Redox Signal. 2010;12(4):503–35.

147 Measuring in vivo mitophagy.
Mol Cell. 2015;60(4):685–96.

148 Mfn2 deficiency links age-related sarcopenia and impaired autophagy to activation of an adaptive mitophagy pathway.
EMBO J. 2016;35(15):1677–93.

149 Mitochondrial dynamics, mitophagy and cardiovascular disease.
J Physiol. 2016;594(3):509–25.

150 Development of monocytes, macrophages, and dendritic cells.
Science. 327: 656–661

# Neogenesis

151 The placebo effect: illness and interpersonal healing.
Perspect. Biol. Med. 2009 Autumn; 52 (4): 518

152 Weatherman's Guide to the Sun;
Ben Davison, September 1, 2020

153 Prevalence of sarcopenia in the world: a systematic review
and meta- analysis of general population studies
J Diabetes Metab Disord. 2017; 16: 21.

154 The diagnosis of osteoporosis
J Bone Miner Res 9(8):1137–41. 1994.

155 Muse Cells Are Endogenous Reparative Stem Cells
Adv Exp Med Biol; 2018; 1103:43-68.

156 Unique multipotent cells in adult human mesenchymal cell
populations;
*Proceedings of the National Academy of Sciences. 107 (19): 8639–43.*

157 Multilineage-differentiation stress-enduring (Muse) cells
are a primary source of induced pluripotent stem cells in
human fibroblasts
*Proceedings of the National Academy of Sciences. 108 (24): 9875-80.*

158 Muse Cells Provide the Pluripotency of Mesenchymal
Stem Cells: Direct Contribution of Muse Cells to Tissue
Regeneration.
*Cell Transplantation 25 (5): 849-61.*

159 Mobilization of Pluripotent Multilineage-Differentiating
Stress-Enduring Cells in Ischemic Stroke;
Journal of Stroke and Cerebrovascular Diseases. 25 (6): 1473–81.

160 *m*TOR and the health benefits of exercise
Seminars in Cell & Dev. Biology, Vol. 36, Dec. 2014, Pages 130-139

161 The Role of the Anabolic Properties of Plant- versus
Animal-Based Protein Sources in Supporting Muscle Mass
Maintenance: A Critical Review
Nutrients. 2019 Aug; 11(8): 1825.

162 Scientists discover staggering amount of life deep below
Earth's surface
https://astronomy.com/news/2018/12/scientists-discover-staggering-amount-
of- life-deep-within-earth

163 Not by Fire but by Ice: Discover What Killed the
Dinosaurs...and Why It Could Soon Kill Us
Robert Felix; Sugarhouse Pub. Nov. 1, 1999

# Neogenesis

**164 Aging in Reverse: A Review of Counterclockwise**
MIND & BODY Articles & More; SEPTEMBER 25, 2009

**165 Can you trick your ageing body into feeling younger?**
https://www.bbc.com/news/magazine-11284180

**166 Mechanism of Fatty-Acid-Dependent UCP1 Uncoupling in Brown Fat Mitochondria**
Cell. 2012 Oct 12; 151(2): 400–413.

**167 Stress could help activate brown fat**
https://www.sciencedaily.com/releases/2016/02/160208213648.htm

**168 Real-Life Benefits of Exercise and Physical Activity**
https://www.nia.nih.gov/health/real-life-benefits-exercise-and-physical-activity

**169 https://www.youtube.com/watch?v=iC75qSbaGPQ**

**170 Super Fuel: Ketogenic Keys to Unlock the Secrets of Good Fats, Bad Fats, and Great Health;** Dr. **Joseph Mercola** and Dr. **James DiNicolantonio**; **ISBN:** 1401956351

# Neogenesis

Made in United States
North Haven, CT
24 February 2022

16445265R00095